a
common
thread

16 personal accounts of faith, fertility issues, and miscarriage

Compiled and Edited by
Catherine Sylvester

Published in the United States

A Common Thread

Infertility affects one in six couples; and one in four pregnancies will end in miscarriage.

The physical toll is significant, but what of the heart, the head, and the spirit? When author Catherine Sylvester and her husband found themselves on the fertility roller coaster, suffering four miscarriages over two years, she found little to relate to, or to bring comfort, in the bookshops she frequented.

Midway through their journey (between their third and fourth miscarriage) God birthed something else within her heart – a ministry to helps others traversing the same rocky road; Thursday's Babies (www.thursdaysbabies.com).

Through monthly newsletters and regular correspondence with others, Catherine was able to share her story, and to offer hope and honesty to a situation that is so infrequently addressed, yet is so all-consuming to those going through it.

Additionally, the seeds of a book were sown at that time. What would happen if she had a resource that she could place into anyone's hands who was experiencing fertility issues/miscarriage? What would that book look like? No two journeys are the same – some undergo medical intervention, some don't. Some have a medical reason for their difficulties or loss; others do not. The range and scope of problems and issues that arise is enormous. How could one such book be relevant for all? Although we all experience the journey differently, we all share 'a common thread.'

A Common Thread is a collection of brutally honest accounts of fertility issues or miscarriage. Each journey is unique; yet each contributor shares truthfully from their heart the highs and lows they have been through; how their journey has affected their faith and how God has brought them through; the physical, emotional and mental toll it has taken on them; and where they are now.

Catherine's hope is that as each reader moves through the pages, they will be able to relate to different parts of each story.

A Common Thread includes stories of those who have experienced successful IVF, failed IVF, multiple miscarriage, miscarriage after having children, adoption, miracle births and those who have never been able to have children.

For Julian
You are truly everything good rolled into one.
To the moon and back B.W. xx

TABLE OF CONTENTS

Title	Page

<u>Welcome</u>

When I suffered my third miscarriage, I felt terribly alone in my pain. Other than the beautiful *Jesse Found in Heaven* I could not find something in the bookstores to minister to my aching heart. Not only were we experiencing the crushing grief of loss, but were also undergoing fertility treatment in the form of monitored medication. I longed to know I was not on my own during this time. I needed to know that the emotions and questions I was experiencing and asking were not unusual or wrong.

A while later, when Thursday's Babies was born out of a desire to see hope restored where it had seemingly been lost in the area of fertility issues, I believe that God gave me a vision for such a book. This book.

It is not a how-to book. It will not attempt to tell you how to deal with your grief, your losses, your inability to get pregnant as and when you would like. It will not try to mend your relationship with God or offer a sure-fire method for tackling fertility treatment.

My desire is that as you turn the pages and read through others' accounts of fertility issues and loss, you will be able to relate to different parts of different journeys. Even if your circumstances may differ, I hope there will be a deeper recognition within you. For even though all our stories differ somewhat in their details, I believe you will discover we all share a common thread.

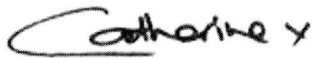

Acknowledgements

My God

Thank you so much, my Heavenly Father and King. You truly are a Redeemer, for you have taken my life from a place of loss and pain to one of joy, love, and purpose. I do not have the words to express my gratitude, so I offer up two simple ones … Thank you.

My husband

I am grateful beyond description that God gave me you as my husband and provision. You make me laugh, you hold me up, you are my best bud and my amazing man. I am so thankful we get to do this together. I couldn't do it without you. I love you. Thank you.

My daughters

Estella June and Skyler Rose, you are both blessings, delights, just incredible. Thank you, thank you, Lord, for our daughters. Custom-made for us by a phenomenal Creator. I love you, my baby girls. Thank you for being ours.

My editor

Oh Jan! Little did we know that first meeting at the café what a great adventure we were embarking on. How do I thank you for investing so much of your heart, your talent, and your patience into this book? You delicately held the vision and gave it such deep respect. From all of us – thank you. Thank you for honoring our words and our journeys. Thank you.

My family

Mum and Dad, Mark and Ann, I love you guys. You are wonderful and I couldn't have yummier parents or in-laws. Thank you for walking this journey out with us and for holding us up in your prayers. Thank you for being the best grandparents ever. Thank you.

My friends

Karo – spiritual mama, prayer warrior, walking buddy, patient ear, incredible family woman, wise, loving, generous; Libs – fabulous listener, tender heart, gracious woman of God; Meg – choccy pal, my fun-to–be-pregnant-with friend; Sarah – I love ya, you make me laugh; Sammy – fellow traveler; Jo – always smiling, so encouraging; Vetty – I love you, honey. You are truly dear to my heart; Lisa – you are the friend who weeps with those who weep, and who weeps out of joy when there is something to celebrate; Tenielle - love, love you.

You are *all* special. I love you Thank you.

My prayer warriors
I want to thank every person who has ever offered up a prayer for us. Prayer is so powerful; thank you for being strong when we were weary. Thank you, my Thursday's Babies women – you are inspirational. Thank you.

The lovely Pastor Chris
You are so generous in every way – your time, your heart, your friendship. Thank you for loving us instantly and for celebrating with us wholeheartedly. Thank you.

Matt and Kaleena
Thank you so very, very much for blessing us. The few hours of work you offered to do for us turned into a few years! You *know* I couldn't do the technological website things without you (see, even that sentence is so untechnological!!) Thank you.

Tracey
Thank you for your generosity in sharing your knowledge of all things booky with me! In birthing this baby you are the doula when the pushing got tiring. Thank you.

* * *

This book is dedicated to every person out there battling fertility issues, infertility, and loss. It is my prayer that through these pages, you will discover a granule or two of hope and encouragement. I also pray that through these brave and honest accounts of others' journeys, you will catch more than a glimpse of the overwhelming, awesome love that a great and Heavenly Father holds in His heart for you.

You are not alone.

You are loved.

Forward

My friendship with Catherine began simply—with "a common thread." I had suffered the loss of a baby in the womb in the early 1970's. And Catherine, a young, vibrant woman with her own story of loss, had come across my little book, *Jesse Found in Heaven*, and was touched. From there, our connection of encouragement began.

At the time--with the promise of a healthy birth still an unfulfilled dream in her heart, I was drawn to Catherine's contagious optimism and delightful spirit of faith for others. I admired her compassion and loved the fact that she was helping so many through her "Thursday's Babies" newsletters. She was encouraging, believing, informing, and connecting with those whose experiences could be expressed in their own voices, in a safe place where they would be heard.

When I met Catherine and her husband Julian in Sydney, they were believing to conceive, again. We joined in prayer and outside that little cafe, we shared a clear sense they would hold a "bonny" baby in their arms! Sure enough, they conceived and are now the proud parents of adorable wee Estella and Skyler!

As you will discover, Catherine's book is the story of her influence on the lives of other women to never give up in the face of adversity... to worship the Lord in the midst of the storm... to find strength in female friendship, and to cleave to the absolute that "God is Good" no matter what the circumstance.

May you find the story you need to find... meet the women you need to meet... hear the words you so need to hear, and see the God who sees and loves you so.

Big Hugs always xxx Chris

Chris Pringle - Senior Pastor
C3 Church Oxford Falls
Sydney, Australia

a
common
thread

REDEEMED

Catherine's Story

"I will redeem this."

As I sat on the couch, tears streaming down my face, anger boiling up inside me, this gentle word from God tenderly touched my spirit, bringing a glimmer of hope. I had just returned home from an ultrasound at the seventh week of my pregnancy.

Only one week previously we had caught a glimpse of the tiniest flutter of a heartbeat. Today – nothing. Our baby had died. Our third miscarriage was imminent.

A year earlier, in February 2006, my husband Julian and I had embarked on one of the most exciting adventures of our lives – the quest to get pregnant. Little did we know it would take twenty-five months of disappointment, nine rounds of the fertility drug Clomiphene (Clomid), and four miscarriages before we would become pregnant with our first miracle baby, Estella.

We had no idea those two years would be filled with the highest of highs and the lowest of lows. Our hope would be all but annihilated, as month after month the desire of our hearts remained unmet, out of reach. Like so many couples, it had never occurred to us that we would not be able to conceive when we liked. We had no idea that statistics show it is not uncommon for couples to try for up to a year before being successful.

There are no guarantees that the way we see things playing out will be what eventually happens. It calls to mind Proverbs 16:9

(MSG), "We plan the way we want to live, but only GOD makes us able to live it."

The first time we actively tried to conceive, I assumed that right then, in that very moment, I could indeed be pregnant. I would phone Julian on my lunch breaks at work, just to remind him of this fact. I am smiling as I write this. I am smiling at the pure innocence of our hearts. That we had no concept of what was ahead of us is an understatement. We were just so thrilled the time had come to expand our family to more than me and him and the cat!

That is one of the things fertility issues rob people of—the pure, joyful spontaneity of starting a family. Our daydreams of future pregnancies never once included multiple blood tests, internal ultrasounds, specimen collections, scans, specialist appointments, fertility drugs with awful side effects, or loss. Even if it took us a few months to conceive, I assumed the first medical professional we saw would be the midwife, not the fertility doctor! The move from natural to clinical was relatively subtle, until one day we woke up and were knee-deep in chromosomal translocations and falling HCG levels.

When we married in October 2005, I had chosen the natural fertility method of contraception, which involves temperature taking and looking for signs of ovulation. I became very in tune with my cycle, so I was fairly certain our timing was accurate. It was more than a little disappointing when months ticked by and nothing was happening.

In May 2006 I believe I got pregnant. My charting and temperature taking confirmed I was quite late, but even before I took a pregnancy test I miscarried. Two further miscarriages at a similar stage were the same—quite different from a missed period.

Every month that passed was a roller coaster. The first two weeks were filled with the lows of disappointment and sadness, then from the middle of the month, hope started to rise—the "what ifs"—only to be dashed. Then the roller coaster would start again. I read all I could, took every basic blood test available, and even had an ultrasound to ensure everything was healthy. I took folic acid—

so many months of folic acid —and pregnancy multivitamins. But still nothing.

In November 2006, although we hadn't yet been trying for a year, deep in my heart I knew something was wrong. I recall praying one day, trying unsuccessfully to avoid the "Why, God? Why not us?" questions, when I felt the Holy Spirit's prompting - "It's a spiritual battle." Little did I know this truth would become increasingly important on the journey to the redemption of our fertility issues.

From then on I began to pray in a different way for our children. I began to go to battle for them. We also decided it was time to get ourselves checked out from a more specialized medical point of view.

Julian and I visited a fertility clinic. They ran a battery of tests, all of which came back clear. I started on clomiphene (Clomid) to ensure I was producing some healthy eggs each month. On our first cycle we conceived. This was our first officially confirmed pregnancy. Our joy was overwhelming.

The clinic closely monitored my HCG levels (the hormone that indicates a continuing pregnancy). Each of their phone calls was more disappointing than the first as my levels dropped and I miscarried our longed-for baby.

Life goes on between tests, hoping, and praying. Between learning we were pregnant and losing that baby, Julian turned thirty-one and his grandfather passed away. During every moment of dealing with our lives I was worrying and hoping and calling the clinic. Those were very long days.

As heartbroken as we were, at last we felt we were in good medical hands. My doctor ordered tests for recurrent miscarriage. I now see the blessing in these tests, because technically they are only undertaken after three officially recorded miscarriages. I am so grateful she ordered these tests when she did, as the results produced an answer to our questions—Julian has a balanced chromosomal translocation. Although this doesn't affect him in any way, it can have a serious effect on conceiving and maintaining a pregnancy.

At the time of these tests my work required us to live in a different city from our fertility specialist. What's more, we needed a genetic counselor, who lived and worked in yet another city, to explain the condition. It was a few weeks until we could get an appointment at her monthly clinic in our hometown. More waiting.

A few days after our diagnosis we found out I was pregnant again. We couldn't wait to discover what it all meant, so that Saturday we took a ten-hour round trip to see the genetic counselor, who kindly gave up her morning for us.

Sitting in her office, in a maternity hospital of all places, felt quite surreal. I had a strange sense of excitement. Excitement that we were actually going to get some answers about why we had miscarried and what we would be facing in our endeavours to have a baby.

The counselor was wonderful. She had charts and printouts and gave us all the information we needed. She explained a relatively complicated condition in plain terms. She even gave us copies to give to our extended family so they could understand our situation as well.

I couldn't do justice to the description of a translocation here, but in a nutshell it was really just "luck of the draw" how the sperm cell split and whether we would get a "good" split or not. If we got a "bad" split we would most likely miscarry before twelve weeks. For reasons they are not sure of, it sometimes means conception can be difficult too. And finally, there is *absolutely nothing* the doctors can do to fix it.

With our tiny six-week-old fetus on board and more than a little shell shocked, we took the long drive home. I was acutely aware that it would be very easy for Julian to take the issue all on himself and feel responsible for the situation. It was extremely important to me that we allow no room for blame. We talked everything through. I made it clear to Julian that what had happened in his body was not his fault in the slightest, and ultimately God is in control. I didn't lay blame on him and I hoped he wouldn't either.

There is nothing like being told medicine can't help to make you realize serious prayer is in order. I pleaded with God for the life inside me. Seeing the fluttering heartbeat of our baby reassured me greatly, but within days the blood tests showed my HCG levels were doing some strange and unusual things. They had risen, but not enough. It became difficult over the next week to get a straight answer from any of the local doctors or blood labs. I was continually told to wait and see, which was an excruciating prospect.

During this time I needed to keep on working. My job entailed quite long hours, and in my role I couldn't hide in a corner and cry – although I did take many trips to the bathroom to do so.

I was open with the two colleagues who shared my workspace, and my immediate manager, who was new to the role, became my own personal sounding board. Her support and kindness truly helped me get through those long days of waiting.

I struggled to stay focused on the task at hand as I battled fear and constantly checked that my pregnancy symptoms were still there. A friend referred to my constant wing-like arm maneuvers to check for breast tenderness as my "chicken dance."

I desperately wanted someone, anyone, to tell me everything was going to be okay. I wanted God to confirm the life inside me would survive. I ached for just one doctor to give me a trace of hope. But there was only a deafening silence until our seven-week scan when our baby was no more. We were devastated.

A dear friend wisely gave me space to download my grief and anger over a long phone call. The opportunity to pour out every confused, painful emotion without someone trying to fix it for me was such a gift. While in that moment I was not feeling particularly faith-filled, she knew my feet were planted on solid ground and my heart would recover. She knew God was big enough to take it and what I needed was a loving ear. I needed to get it all out. I am forever grateful for that conversation.

Throughout our entire journey Julian has been a rock. What could have driven us apart actually drew us closer together. We leaned on one another in sadness, clung together in hope, and pointed each other to God for true healing and the strength to get through. I am so grateful he is my man.

As I sat on that couch after hanging up the phone, I felt God say, "I will redeem this." Although the broken, hurt part of me wanted to yell back, "but I want my baby!!" something much deeper stirred and my spirit pricked up its ears. The embers of hope were fanned and I felt the crackle of a fire ignite.

I read Genesis 50:19-20 (NIV), where Joseph is reunited with his brothers years after they betrayed him by selling him into slavery. Filled with remorse, they beg his forgiveness. Joseph says to them, "Don't be afraid. Am I in the place of God? You intended to harm me, but God intended it for good to accomplish what is now being done, the saving of many lives." I felt God whisper to me, "What was intended for harm, I will use for good. For the saving of many lives." The crackle became a flame.

I clung to the scripture that all things are possible for God (Matthew 19:26). I elected not to have a D and C, but to allow space for a miracle. As much as I feared losing our baby, I was more fearful of God choosing not to step in to save the situation. How would I cope with the knowledge that all things are possible for God, but sometimes all things are not done by God?

So many of my default settings were negative. I feared God but not in the positive, biblical sense. I was just plain afraid of Him. I found it easy to believe in His promises and His love for other people, but believed everything He wanted to teach me had to be done the hard way, through tough lessons. I wrote in my journal that I didn't want to feel that way, but I didn't know how to change it; only He could.

What would eventually be a two-and-a-half-year journey of healing my relationship with God began then and there. The big issue for me was my disbelief in the goodness of God. I didn't trust Him or His love for me. I knew there was an incredible relationship I could have with my Creator that I wasn't experiencing, and I didn't know how to remedy it. But as so often is the way with God, it turns out I wasn't the one who had to fix it. He had it all covered!

* * *

Sometimes people with good intentions unintentionally said quite hurtful things. "God must've wanted your babies in heaven" and "It's probably all for the best" were recurring themes. Probably the most frequent was "God works good through all things." The truth of this scripture brought little comfort when we lost a longed-for baby. Sometimes people are uncomfortable with grief and feel the need to offer platitudes in an attempt to solve the problem, when nothing other than "I'm sorry" really seems to work. They can't fix the problem, as it's not their problem to fix.

Whether losing a baby through miscarriage or struggling to get pregnant, compassion can be a wonderful thing to receive. Who knows the whys of God? Certainly not me. And most likely not anyone else I know, either. It was those dear people in my life who just listened...and listened...and listened; who held me as I cried; who prayed faith-filled prayers when I had none left to offer up; who walked day to day with me; who never gave up hope for us, I am most thankful for. They made the journey bearable.

* * *

In the three weeks between the seven-week scan and actually miscarrying, God felt very close. I wrote in my journal: "Of course there is a loss. A loss of this pregnancy, a loss of October 18 being a date of joyful delivery, and a loss of this child and the dreams for this child. But within that there is a tiny birth. A birth of hope. The hope of healing. Healing in my relationship with my Father, healing from old and incorrect thoughts and beliefs. A healing of faith."

Some of the most special times for me were within worship. As I sang, I felt God so close to me. I knew He could see there were days when it truly was a sacrifice of praise. There was hardly a time I didn't cry as I sang. He poured His healing balm over me, and I wept and praised and died to myself.

On Sunday, March 25, 2007 my journal records: "On Friday morning our very precious baby went home to Jesus... I feel sad our baby's gone, but we will see her one day."

7

Around this time I was given a book. Pastor Chris Pringle's *Jesse Found in Heaven* reminded me that the babies we miscarry are being raised in heaven. There were days when I stamped my spiritual foot at God getting to raise so many of them instead of us; days when this didn't comfort me as much as I would have liked. But deep down I know these babies are real. They aren't just fetuses or something without purpose and personality. They will never feel pain, be sick, or be separated from God because He, the most perfect parent there is – our heavenly Father – is raising them.

* * *

My work contract completed, we moved back to our home city, nearer our friends and family. I took some time off, as I was exhausted in every way – physically, emotionally, and spiritually. I adored staying home and taking care of us. Every nesting instinct brewing for the past year and a half came out in full force as I experimented with new recipes and made our home a warm place of rest.

I started walking for an hour a day and praying. I would chitchat with God while I walked, then when I got home I would open up the Bible to discover revelation and exciting promises. It was such a special time of communicating with God – listening to Him too, rather than just me speaking.

Reading over my journals from that time, I see my mind was often on the question of where God was calling us next. Both Julian and I felt it was into more ministry endeavors. I had assumed it would be with his playing – as a musician he had been involved with leading worship in various bands for years. Now I see God had other things in mind.

After hearing of another friend miscarrying, I got mad. While out on one of my big God-walks, the words I heard over a year before kept ringing in my ears: "It's a spiritual battle." I raced home and looked up every scripture relating to God's will towards us having children. I was amazed there were so many; some I had never encountered before. I was so excited. The flame ignited at the time of our third miscarriage suddenly burst into a bush fire! I drew up a letter and sent it to all the women I knew who were having issues with conceiving or carrying a child to term. In part it read:

Hi my friend ...

It's funny when God speaks to you isn't it? When I went for my walk this morning, what was really heavy on my heart was the issue of babies. Not just mine, but friends battling infertility and miscarriage.

About a year ago God showed me we are in a battle for the next generation of Christians to rise up and take their place in His army, in His kingdom, in His church. The enemy is not nearly as keen as we are to see this happen. Hence, I believe we are seeing a number of Christian women battling to get pregnant and carry healthy, vibrant babies to term, ready to be raised in the house of God.

For quite some time I have been fasting and praying one day a week about Julian and me having children. You are aware of our struggles with it. As I was walking and praying today, I felt a few ideas come to me. Hopefully they are Holy Spirit inspired, but I know they line up biblically, so they can't be bad!

Imagine what would happen if an army of princess warriors stood up to fight; if modern day Deborahs and Jaels (two women in the book of Judges) drove a peg through the enemy's temple. What damage we could do to the devil's plans for our kids!

*The Bible says when "two of you on earth agree about **anything** you ask for, it will be done for them by my Father in heaven" (Matthew 18:19, NIV). And that "one man can chase a thousand, or two put ten thousand to flight" (Deuteronomy 32:30, NIV).*

God says children are a heritage, a gift, a legacy, a reward (Psalm 127), a blessing He bestows upon us.

I truly believe we will see miracles as we stand and fast and pray together, agreeing on what the Bible says.

It's time to get tough on the enemy, fervent in prayer, united as one under the blood of Christ, claiming our inheritance.

I have fasted and prayed on Thursdays for quite a while. I would love it if you would join me. If you don't want to fast fully, perhaps you would consider joining me in prayer, or doing a mini fast, or whatever you feel led to do...

My vision is to see an army of women standing firm together in victory.

Thursday's Babies was born.

* * *

Since then I have discovered that I was not the first person to stumble on this revelation—that God has put much in His Word about children being a blessing to us from Him! But at the time I had never read anything along these lines and was full of excitement and hope.

One of the overwhelming feelings I struggled with in trying unsuccessfully to get and stay pregnant was powerlessness. It didn't really matter what I did, what vitamins I ingested, what fertility drugs I was prescribed, there was nothing I could do.

But pray! And stand on God's Word. At last I could do something. Deep in my heart I knew it was ultimately up to God. He is the creator of life. No matter our methods, it is in His hands whether or not He breathes being into form. The fine line I have always wrestled with, the delicate balancing act, is whether to leave it all in God's hands, do nothing, or do something in between the two.

* * *

Psalm 127:3-5 (NIV) says, "Sons are a heritage from the Lord, children a reward from him... Blessed is the man whose quiver is full of them. **They will not be put to shame...**"

Sadly it would seem that so many people whose "quivers" are not full, do feel this sense of shame. The well-known chapter with the b-word (barren) in it, Isaiah 54 states that the barren woman will have many children and should not be afraid, for she "will not suffer shame... You will forget the shame of your youth." Again barrenness and shame are linked. I became aware that for many people this was debilitating. They would retreat inwardly, concealing their feelings and hiding from those around them the pain they were in. It broke my heart. There is no shame with the Lord. What if this issue was brought out into the light? Would it help others to share their struggles with loved ones?

I had the opportunity to discuss Thursday's Babies in an interview I gave on national radio, and also to mention it in an article about our journey I wrote for a magazine.

As I spoke about us, I hoped it would be a freeing thing for other people too.

* * *

Riding high on hope, revelation, and a sense of actually being able to do something, in October 2007 I was beyond excited to discover I was pregnant again. I was so sure this would be it. Everything I had learned, everything I now knew about God's plans for having children would surely mean victory, success, and a baby for us! At home on my own, I took the pregnancy test then jumped in the car to deliver the precious stick to Julian at work.

We jumped around like little kids and quickly figured out our due date. No matter how many times we miscarried, it was always one of the first things we did.

Julian will be the first to say it was different for him this time too. He had been "hedging his bets" previously, believing we'd get pregnant but guarding his heart in case we miscarried. But now he was on board 100%.

Now we were pregnant again, I was speaking God's Word out left, right, and center; battling fear and praying hard.

It is an understatement to say we were shocked when I started to bleed some time later. Surely this was not in the plan. It certainly wasn't in *my* plan, but it would appear God's plan was slightly different. I did another pregnancy test and the beautiful positive sign was nowhere to be seen. Just a dark, ugly minus sign. I was minus a baby. Again.

Standing in the bathroom staring in the mirror in shock, tears flowing, I felt God say to me, "Sweetheart, I need you to do this for me." Now I don't usually hear God say things like "sweetheart." It's just not quite the vernacular He seems to use in conversing with me!

At first I thought he meant I needed to battle through in prayer and believe for a miracle. But as I started to bleed more heavily, I couldn't help wondering if He meant I needed to go through this for Him so I could understand His healing love and faithfulness in this area of loss. That sometimes, no matter how many scriptures you stand on and how much you pray and believe, God is still God and only He knows His reasons why things don't always work out in the way we would like best.

Julian stepped up to the plate, wrapped me in his arms, and began to thank God for our babies to come. Then he put on some worship music and we praised God. I truly believe that right there he set the tone for us.

The next few months were bleak for me, as I wrote in my journal at the end of November: "I've been so quiet with God lately. In some ways my faith is so much deeper than ever before, and yet in some ways I feel like I've got cataracts on my heart. Knowing He CAN do anything, yet sometimes chooses NOT to. Feeling afraid to hope."

Throughout our journey there were times of joy when friends announced the great news they were expecting. Hidden deep inside were the times when such news made us so sad that we weren't the ones shouting from the rooftops about our impending birth. Inexplicably it was easy to be around some people's children, while around others jealousy and bitterness would well up. There was no rhyme or reason as to when or why this occurred, and it had absolutely nothing to do with the children or the parents personally.

Family holidays, Christmas in particular, were especially difficult. Each year we wished the next festive season would see our children playing beneath the tree, unwrapping presents, running around with their cousins. It became more difficult to feign enthusiasm for the occasion, so the Christmas after our fourth miscarriage we opted to stay home. We had a small lunch with my parents, and it was an incredible release to enjoy the day rather than having to act happy and joyful.

As 2008 rolled around we began to ponder seriously just how long we would be able – emotionally – to keep on trying. How many miscarriages were we willing to go through in our attempts to expand our family? Isaiah 46:4 (NIV) brought me great strength at this time: "Even to your old age and gray hairs I am he who will sustain you. I have made you and I will carry you; I will sustain you and I will rescue you."

Sustaining and rescuing were very much needed. For various reasons, not everyone in scripture received the promises they were given. Hebrews 11:39 (NIV) makes this clear: "These were all commended for their faith, yet not one of them received what had been promised."

When I started Thursday's Babies, the desire to have hope and something to contribute towards us successfully carrying a child to term spurred me on. Now I was faced with the fact that not everyone who does these things will receive the answer to their prayers in the way they initially had hoped. My heart turned more and more towards the journey for people, rather than just the outcome.

The newsletters I sent out began to focus on the heart and the battering it takes within the journey. Having faith along the way was important and my correspondence with women linked to the ministry was so fulfilling.

By February 2008 I was at the end of myself. I had boxed my way around in spiritual circles and I was spent. With nothing left to pray I merely stood in agreement with Julian's prayers, knowing they would cover me. Leaning on Jesus was my only viable option if I didn't want the pain to take me out of the race.

Everything we had tried in our own strength – the prayers, the fasting, the fertility drugs, the natural treatments – had come to nothing tangible. God was my answer. He would either choose to create and sustain life inside me or not. What had consumed me for two years was not going to destroy me.

I let it go, I exhaled, I released it all to the One who loves me beyond words. The way I carried it out may not have been gracious or pretty, but I relinquished the controls entirely.

I had a vision one night as I drifted in and out of sleep. It was of the woman with the issue of blood. She was me. Moving through the dirty, dusty streets Jesus walked, following a crowd of people trying to get close to the Messiah, I could smell the air and hear the sounds.

At that precise moment I lunged forward and grabbed the hem of His cloak. It was thick, rough hessian. I knew He was the only answer. He is the same Jesus today as He was in biblical times. He turned around, and with nothing but love He asked who had touched him. When I said "me," He smiled warmly and reassuringly. I felt so much love it was incredible.

Surely the woman in the Bible must have tried everything in her twelve years of dealing with bleeding issues. Mark 5:26 (NIV) says "she had suffered a great deal under the care of many doctors and had spent all she had, yet instead of getting better she grew worse."

Sounds similar to that experienced by those in a fertility journey to me! She must have prayed, sought wise counsel, and fasted. Yet when it came down to it, her only answer was Jesus and His power. The same was true for me. I was struggling to keep my head above water, nearly drowning in my grief. It is always darkest before the dawn.

First Corinthians 10:13 (NRSV) states: "God is faithful, and he will not let you be tested beyond your strength, but with the testing he will also provide the way out so that you may be able to endure it." God truly was, and is, my way out when my strength could go no further.

I had signed up for a major women's conference I now had little interest in attending. I am so grateful I did. Louie Giglio preached his "Indescribable" message there. Part of the message goes into the intricacies of life in the womb. Seeing those little babies at the stages I had lost mine was too much for me to bear. I absolutely broke down and cried. I sobbed. I am glad I was surrounded by hundreds of women and not men!

Immediately following the pictures of the babies, he started to address those who felt the bottom had dropped out of life for them.

He began to speak life into broken hearts. He began to explain how very much God loves us. How much He loves me.

I had so desperately needed to hear that. Throughout all the trials and tribulations of fertility treatment and loss, I had truly wondered if God really did love me as He said. For if He did, how could He allow life to go on with so much pain in it?

In that half hour sitting in a great company of women, hearing God's love spoken about, the Holy Spirit stitched up my heart and put fresh bandages on it. It was medicine for my soul.

I knew 100% that this amazing God who created something as huge as the heavens and as intricate as new life loved me. He cared for me. His thoughts towards me were for good and not for harm – no matter how circumstances may have looked to my human eyes. He loved me. He loved me. He loved me. I felt so free. The unbearable burden was lifted.

Within three days I conceived.

* * *

I would like to say that the rest of the road was simple. That once I was pregnant with my daughter, all fears were abandoned and I sat awash in God's loving embrace. But in reality I had to battle fear every step of the way in my pregnancy.

Looking back, it was an ideal nine months, physically. Not a problem at all. Due to our losses we were able to receive specialist care and had scans every week from seven to twelve, then four more after that. It is truly amazing to hold my daughter now and know I have seen her at seven weeks gestation, her heart beating, limbs forming.

Again I rested on Romans 3:4-5 (NIV) that assures me God's faithfulness is not dependent on my human weaknesses. "What if some do not have faith? Will their lack of faith nullify God's faithfulness? Not at all!" Julian's prayers and those of friends buoyed me up and we moved forward.

On December 3, 2008, Estella June entered the world.

She is amazing. An incredible blessing from an incredible Creator. The Lord continues healing my heart. Only recently, as I sat praying, I heard Him whisper into my being the verse from Song of Songs 8:5 (NIV), "Who is this coming up from the desert leaning on her lover?" It is me, it is me.

In the past two and a half years God has done an incredible work in my life. What I strongly suspected at the time of our third miscarriage turned out to be true. He was most interested in mending my relationship with Him and ensuring I had a true and accurate perception of who He is and how He feels towards me.

A culmination of all the events and revelations mentioned here, and so many more that can wait to be told another time, have meant His work has been done in me without my even realizing it fully – till now. I cannot thank Him enough. There are no words to express entirely how amazing it feels to be free.

The Lord is still redeeming our losses, as He promised He would. This book is the fruition of a dream He planted in my heart in the middle of 2007. He has planted other seeds He has watered and they are starting to bloom. He does truly know the plans He has for us, and is working them out according to His purposes and timing, so the glory is His.

As you read this, please know the Lord loves you desperately. No matter the circumstances surrounding your life right now, He knows and He cares. Nothing is beyond redemption.

A year later... In September of 2010, we were incredibly blessed to give birth to our second amazing daughter, Skyler Rose. We are so grateful. She was conceived on our second attempt, without any fertility drugs. Yet another miracle from our miraculous God.

LOVING ACCEPTANCE

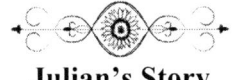

Julian's Story

I grew up in a family that placed great value on time together. With two younger sisters, I had always pictured future family gatherings with my own kids and their cousins playing, having fun, and I looked forward to the opportunity to walk in my father's footsteps of being an awesome dad. Little did I know that this ideal picture was not going to be as easy to achieve as I had first assumed.

Catherine and I met in our early thirties and late twenties, respectively. Between us we had lived fairly transient lives, following our dreams. At first we were in no hurry to start a family; we figured that when we were ready we would get pregnant and would move into that new chapter of our lives easily. As it turned out, our being ready had little to do with the situation.

After just four months of marriage we both suddenly felt it was time to extend our team of two to three. Over the next two years we went through four miscarriages, had various appointments with different doctors, specialists, nutritionists, physiotherapy, and even a genetic counselor. It certainly wasn't the "okay, let's start a family" experience I had originally imagined.

Catherine became pregnant after a few months of trying but miscarried at an early stage. She felt strongly that there was something not quite right so we went to see a fertility specialist. We were instructed to undertake a series of tests to check if there were any issues. Thankfully, everything was fine. Particularly for me, much to my relief as a man, my "swimmers" were more than capable of reaching the finish line.

So we left our appointment armed with some new rules, like reducing my coffee intake, increasing exercise, etc., as these things would apparently help our cause. Catherine was also put on a fertility drug (clomiphene/Clomid) to help improve the chance of conception, as the specialist felt some assistance wouldn't hurt. I also learned that as far as conceiving was concerned that there was "a window" of time in which we needed to "plant the seed." This took some getting used to, as our sex life now was dictated by the calendar. It didn't help that I played in a band based in a city a two-hour flight from where we lived. I was also touring for three to four weeks at a time, four or five times a year, which meant I wasn't always in the right place at the right time.

To our joy, reducing coffee, exercising, and the fertility drugs paid off and the next month Catherine was pregnant, but sadly, she miscarried again. Our doctor ordered some more in-depth tests to be done due to the fact that we were now entering "Recurrent Miscarriage" territory.

As a husband this was interesting to deal with, as physically it was Catherine who had to experience all the drugs and early stage of pregnancy and miscarriage. I felt there was not a lot I could do to help her. It was particularly difficult that the whole fertility journey was so absorbing and all-consuming for her. It was her body, her hormones experiencing it all, but for me it was different. It was important, of course, but not as intense. Additionally, the fertility drug she was on greatly affected her moods. There were highs and lows and everything in between. It was especially painful for her, as she naturally connected with the baby even at the early stages. To have now lost two, was difficult, to say the least. At times all I could do was hold her tight and just be with her. Words couldn't fix it, but supporting her and being there for her was what she needed.

A couple of months later we were in different cities due to our work commitments. I was in Auckland staying on a friend's couch, attending band rehearsals and preparing for a music festival; Catherine was meeting me the following week.

On a lunch break I received a phone call from the doctor to inform me that the in-depth blood test results were in and there was a problem showing up with mine. She told me I have what's called a balanced translocation. It is a genetic condition that doesn't affect me personally (some friends would beg to differ!). It is either passed on genetically or happens at conception. The specialist informed me that although I'm not affected day to day by the condition, there are a number of different problems it can cause when trying to conceive and carry a baby. These conditions vary from making conception difficult, to causing miscarriage, to major birth defects. She advised me that we would need to see a genetic counselor to determine the severity of my condition and what it could mean for our plans to have a family. Suddenly my previous relief of being fine left me. I instantly felt the weight and responsibility of what we had been going through.

This was quite a bombshell. I had to face the fact that our problems were seemingly "my fault." To add to the pressure, there was a chance Catherine was pregnant. I now knew these test results … and she didn't. I felt conflicted. Should I call and tell her over the phone what I had just found out? Or would it cause her stress, which wouldn't help if she was pregnant? Or should I wait until we were together to talk it through? I decided to wait until I saw her in person.

The next few days were tough. Catherine and I would talk everyday on the phone, and I had to keep this from her. Meanwhile, I was lying on my friend's couch at night, thinking through all the "what ifs" and "whys?" In some ways it was good to know why we were having problems, but there were still many unanswered questions and a feeling of guilt that it was my fault.

Catherine arrived and I picked her up at the airport. We attended the music festival and that night when we sat down at the hotel, I filled her in on the news I had received. To be honest I don't remember a lot about how the conversation went or her reaction, other than it immediately drew us closer together. We both felt some amount of relief that at least we now knew why we were having problems.

Catherine didn't at this stage, nor any other stage, lay any blame on me, which was very humbling. I did, however, initially lay a lot on myself, feeling that these difficulties were due to me. Ultimately and after time, I knew it was completely out of my control and there was nothing I could do about it. Realizing this did help me deal with it somewhat, but didn't change the hardest thing, which was seeing my best friend in so much pain, both emotional and physical as a result. As it turned out, about six days after I received the phone call informing me of the condition, we found out that Catherine was indeed pregnant again.

This was exciting but also scary, knowing about the balanced translocation, which could cause complications. Complications we had yet to have explained fully to us. Because it's a relatively specialized topic, we had to drive for five hours to attend the appointment with a genetic counselor, as there weren't any in the city where we lived.

We learned that each time we got pregnant there was a chance it would be successful, depending on how the chromosomes split. In a nutshell, we just needed to keep trying for as long as we were mentally and emotionally able, until we got "the right split." If we got the "wrong spilt," the fetus would not survive beyond twelve weeks, which could explain our two previous miscarriages.

We also learned there is no cure for the condition and there was nothing we could do physically to improve our chances of getting pregnant and maintaining the pregnancy. The one good thing was that the coffee ban was lifted, as this was not a contributing factor anymore! So we left, picked up a double-shot latte, and embarked on our long drive home, a little shell-shocked and nervous, knowing we already had a baby on board.

Within a few weeks we had a scan and actually saw our baby's heartbeat. This was amazing, as the prior pregnancies had ended before being able to see this. Suddenly this baby was a reality for me and some excitement grew. Part of being in the care of our specialists meant Catherine had blood tests to monitor hormone levels that indicate if the baby is developing and growing at the required rate. These results had been up and down, so the outcome of this baby was in question. Now that we could see a heartbeat though, it was a positive sign and gave us both some much-needed hope. Unfortunately, the levels continued to fluctuate so we had to have another ultrasound. Crushingly, there was no heartbeat.

One of the hardest things about the journey was the ups and downs, highs and lows. One week there was a heartbeat, and the hormone levels were great. The next the levels were going down and no heartbeat. I found when it was looking good I started to get into the headspace of "this is it—we are really going to have our baby." Those thoughts were then dashed as we were told the levels had dropped and so on.

This miscarriage was especially difficult, as it required Catherine to be admitted to the hospital when the bleeding became too heavy. It became particularly real to me this time–up till now, I had never seen anything physical happen. But to hold Catherine's hand as they surgically removed our dead baby from her body, then have it held up to my face by a medical student, excited that it was in one piece, made it so real.

I felt angry that what was so huge and heartbreaking for us was an exciting learning exercise for a student doctor. While Catherine stayed in the hospital that night, I went home and felt completely numb and alone. It was a lot to take in, and even though deep down I knew it wasn't "my fault," I still battled feelings of responsibility and that I was to blame.

By now we were starting to feel the pressure of our journey. I found I didn't always understand some of the things Catherine would be feeling or saying. Occasionally she would have problems socializing with people if kids were going to be there, or she wouldn't want to go to church on Mother's Day.

Although I mostly understood, I don't think I will ever truly grasp the full enormity of those feelings. As a man, my natural tendency was to want to fix it and make it all better. However, I found this wasn't what she really needed. Nor did she require me to explain the whys or hows. What she needed most from me was just to be there. At times I had to let her "vent," even if occasionally I didn't fully understand what she was feeling. Again, to be there to listen and not always offer suggestions but let her know that she was doing well and would be okay were the best things I could do.

Even though it was particularly hard to do, not trying to solve the problem was very important. At times I would gently "guide" her onto a different path of thinking through our conversation, but I would really try to let her get it all out, the good, the bad, and the ugly! I didn't worry that she meant everything she said. I knew her faith was built on solid ground.

In the months to follow we moved back to Auckland and once again Catherine was pregnant. Until then I had had a certain amount of faith that God would give us the desires of our heart but had always limited myself as to how much I would actually believe each pregnancy would be successful. I think this was partly to protect myself from having to question why if it didn't happen. Also, I didn't have an answer for Catherine, who was at times questioning why God wasn't appearing to answer our prayers. I was now at the point though, of feeling "enough is enough." So we prayed and really believed in faith that this time we would have our baby. It was then a huge shock to us when once again Catherine miscarried.

But this time enough really was enough, and we chose to surround ourselves with worship music. Although we had no idea why we were going through this I still, deep down, believed that God knew the best plan for us. I felt it was time I stepped up, and as the head of our household, I chose to fight for our future babies. I spent some time in rather heated conversations with God and took on more of the spiritual side of our battle than I previously had.

We began to consider how many more times we could go through this. I was getting to the place of thinking we may not ever have kids and although it could be a struggle, I was prepared to trust that for us, that would be God's best plan. This wasn't always easy, as I had such a desire to be a dad, but eventually I came to the place of putting it down and being content with moving on with our lives.

By now it was Christmas 2007. Christmases were tough, because Catherine found it difficult being around all the little ones in my extended family. Even though we loved seeing them, we had thought that by now we would be turning up to enjoy the festivities with our own family. And yet here I was, the eldest of three, and the only one without children of my own. The previous Christmas we had said to each other, "Oh next Christmas we'll have a baby," but it still hadn't come to pass.

As a result we decided to stay in Auckland and not spend Christmas with my family. This was one of the times I didn't completely understand what Catherine was feeling but felt it was really important to allow her the space she needed and protect her from being in a situation that could cause her to be upset and uncomfortable.

We now felt we were coming to the end of what we were able to stand as far as continued miscarriages. Catherine had had enough of taking the fertility drugs that were taking their toll on her emotionally, and I was ready to go for plan B, which was to continue life without kids and trust that we would be fine. Additionally, the striving to have a child really was starting to take over every part of our lives; it was becoming too much. Then in March 2008, Catherine became pregnant. We were very excited, but this time we also decided that if it wasn't successful we would move on with our lives.

As in previous pregnancies, Catherine had lots of blood tests to monitor her hormone levels. After she had taken the test the nurse at the Recurrent Miscarriage Clinic would call with the results.

Catherine didn't want to receive these phone calls herself anymore. I would take them and then relay the info to her. These calls basically told us if the pregnancy would continue. So now for me, it was a very real day-to-day experience.

As to be expected, Catherine would be anxious and worried about the outcome. I would continually be saying "you'll be fine, etc.," but on the inside I had no idea and was freaking out. I had to be strong and reassuring though, to keep her in a good headspace. I was very busy with my job at this time and found work to be a good distraction to take my mind off things during the day. Finally, after many phone calls with results, tears, and prayers, we made it to week seven of the pregnancy. This meant an ultrasound to see our baby, to see her heartbeat. I clearly remember where I was and what I was doing when I got the phone call to say Catherine's levels were fine enough to move on to this important next stage.

It was all quite nerve–wracking, as we had not been this far successfully before. We both were very excited yet had our guards up a little. Personally, throughout the pregnancy, I believed in faith, yet still was not allowing myself to get entirely attached until I was holding that baby. On December 3, 2008, we were very blessed to have Estella June Sylvester make our team of two become three, and I was able to do just that—hold our baby!

I had the absolute joy twenty-one months later of holding our other little miracle, Skyler Rose!

Some people say, "If I had to do it all over again I would, because of the great lessons I've learned." But if I'm honest, I would say I'd rather have just had kids. It wasn't the most fun way to spend the first few years of our marriage, because it was so all-consuming. But then at the same time, those tough few years have proved to be a great foundation-building time for our relationship. So although I wouldn't necessarily choose to go through it again, I can see that there have definitely been some positives come from the experience.

FULLNESS OF LIFE

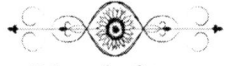

Diane's Story

SITTING in one of our favourite cafés, I glance at a couple of mums, one holding her baby over her shoulder towards me. I think to myself, "what a really lovely baby." But then I find myself daring to imagine what it would feel like to be holding my own little baby, to be out with my friends with their babies. Although enjoying the richness of the moment, moistness again comes to my eyes, so I quickly jump back to reality.

Watching a TV talk show featuring a famous dad with a real gift for putting his emotions into words describing how he feels about his little daughter; the depth of love, the strength of emotion, how he didn't think he could love someone that deeply, I again let my feelings go down that road. This time in the safety and privacy of my lounge, tears well up from that cavernous reality of knowing my husband and I will never experience this.

Enjoying watching my favourite little toddler at church just freely being a toddler, I am reminded of how I looked at that age in photos. Tears well up again because I will never ever see a little piece of my husband and me reflected in our children.

The precious moment captured in a photo of me cradling my pyjama-clad one-year-old niece still so tiny from being born twelve weeks premature, as she falls asleep snuggled into my shoulder. The love I feel for her, the beauty of the well of longing to nurture. It is a small outlet; a photo I look at even now to relive the moment – often with bitter and sweet tears.

Pausing to browse over a selection of books for sale at church and opening an illustrated children's story of Hannah, how she longed to have a baby and how the other women teased and looked down on her.

Looking at the picture of her crying alone away from all the other women, I identify with her pain. Once again I fight back the tears. The pain of infertility is very private.

Being genuinely happy that my good friend and her husband were expecting their first baby, but getting off the phone and bawling my eyes out.

Earlier that day another good friend had phoned to say they were also having a baby. Both friends were my bridesmaids. I had dreamed of sharing being a mum with these two precious women. Then once again hiding the secret pain that my husband and I, after meeting and marrying at age thirty-two, have been secretly trying for a baby for some time.

These are just some of the secret moments I have. Moments I now treasure, because they are a part of my story. They are a part of who I am.

* * *

The pain of not being able to welcome a baby into our world, despite feeling perfectly ready and prepared, is a pain so hard to process, let alone to share with those we live life with day to day. I was no newcomer to the reality that sometimes "bad things happen to good people and sometimes good things happen to bad people". I knew the ability to have babies was not a matter of fairness or deservedness, or even a reflection of one's ability to be a "good" parent. Even so, at times I began blaming myself, thinking this was my fault. And although never doubting God's goodness, I did feel it was I who was perhaps just not quite good enough.

We both felt that adoption wasn't for us. We had our heart set on a biological baby of our own. We wanted to bring so much joy to those around us with a new little life. We wanted to carry on the family name. My husband is his parents' only son, so it was up to us to do this for them. We dreamed of the moment of introducing our baby to a growing number of cousins and the delight they would find in this new little one. We dreamed of names and how we would raise this child, of how it would change our lifestyle. We dreamed of teaching and showing our little one the fun and exciting adventures of life in our world. But this was not to be.

Initially we were quite stunned by it all. We decided not to have any medical investigations. We didn't want fertility treatments, so there was no point. Nothing can explain the turmoil of not knowing, of each month feeling the hormonal and physical highs of hoping we would be pregnant, the increasing mood swings, of being so in tune with every little change in my body and living carefully so as to not harm a possible pregnancy, only to come crashing down each month into the valley of disappointment and despair.

During this phase people started to realize that something was not going to plan, so all the "helpful" advice came along. Some received our choice not to have investigations with anger. Some interpreted our lack of tests and treatment as indicative of us not really desperately wanting to be parents. They were so wrong. Even though we were wrestling with infertility without treatment, we wanted a baby just as much as a couple who takes on the most advanced fertility treatments available. Everyone sets limits where they are most comfortable.

At times I vented my anger at my ever-patient husband and wondered whether we should perhaps get some medical help. I felt I couldn't handle the turmoil any longer. I was angry. I was hurt. I was trying to carry on my normal life working in a job I'd really had enough of and had expected to leave to be a mum. Instead I had to watch many of my workmates live my dream instead. I was not coping that well.

The strange thing is that when we needed the support so badly, it was just too private and too hard for us to understand, let alone share with others. It still breaks my heart to think how many couples go through this without someone to understand and hear their pain.

As we continued on we eventually felt able to share our journey of pain with more people around us. One couple we shared with continue to be such great support. It was a privilege to celebrate the arrival of their just-as-longed-for first baby during this time. They sensitively included us in their joy. In fact ours was the first house their little son visited as a newborn! As it turned out, we were able to share their journey of pain, when they had to adjust their dreams for their lovely son when he was diagnosed as having special needs. Our pain of infertility has created opportunities of privilege to be part of other people's journeys that are painful as well.

We accepted the reality that it didn't look likely we would be parents. However we were never able to totally let that hope go. We enjoyed life together and made plans for the future; plans that included me leaving work for a time because I *chose* to, as I realized I didn't need to have a baby to do this.

I began going for little runs to get fit and have now done four marathons and eight half marathons. This has been a great outlet for anger and stress. It has been good weight control and something I could achieve that required much mental strength, particularly since I'm not naturally athletic. Running the last few kilometers of the marathons became quite a spiritual experience for me as I pushed my body and mind to persevere in the face of mental and physical agony. Running is also something I could not easily do while carrying a baby or even caring for young children.

* * *

In September 2006 we received a letter that was to change our infertility journey forever. It is the part of the journey I still enjoy celebrating. It said, "This is to confirm that I have booked you for publicly funded IVF treatment..."

You see, earlier, when I was thirty-nine, after almost five long years of moving on with our lives but still hoping, we had decided to have a few basic tests done after all, just to see if perhaps there was an obvious cause for our infertility before I turned the big 4-0. At that time we still had the intention of not really embarking on any major intervention. We decided to have a private consultation with a fertility specialist.

This was the result of us having processed our journey a lot more deeply; this time from a situation of greater contentment, having really accepted who we were as a couple and being child-free. Of significance was that I had left my job and we had relocated to a bigger city so my husband could undertake theological studies as part of his response to a strong impression that God had called him many years ago to become a minister. Part of his studies involved a major research project on "The Trauma of Being Human," for which he had chosen to study infertility. We really had gotten to a place where life was very good.

We had gone to see the specialist a month before I turned forty, only to find out that for any publicly funded treatment I *had* to be on the waiting list *before* turning forty. After a discussion the specialist applied for funding in case we decided to have any interventions. In one month's time I would not have been eligible.

That is how we came to receive the letter of confirmation. After walking around our little flat reading and rereading it, we felt there was no reason to turn it down. God could be in this and was well able to "close the door" if that was what He considered best for us.

More appointments followed for the IVF, including a plan of PGD (pre-genetic diagnosis) involving biopsy of a three-day-old embryo at about the eight-cell stage, to test one or two cells for a specified chromosomal disorder, as we had become aware that a chromosomal translocation might be the cause of our infertility.

Our chromosomal translocation would mean the chance of miscarriage prior to twelve weeks of any achieved pregnancy was incredibly high. The embryos would be tested so the unaffected embryos could be used as priority.

This was HUGE for us. I remember writing in my journal, "I have thought so hard about this that my brain hurts"; the "this" being the bio-ethical and spiritual issues of when life begins. Are we playing God? What would we do if there were any fertilised embryos left over? We came to the conclusion that we would pray that God would not let us go beyond acceptable boundaries for our lives and His best plan. So on we went, not sure what future dilemmas we would need to make decisions about, but trusting Him as we faced them.

By this stage we had long given up on keeping our journey of infertility a secret. We were in a close-knit group of great friends and family, and we shared our journey openly with whoever was gracious enough to listen. Many of our single friends sympathised with our story, simply because they had not yet even had the privilege of meeting their life-long partners to be in an acceptable position to try and have longed-for children. At the time of receiving our IVF letter, I had settled back into my work, but this time I was really enjoying my job. My workmates were brilliant, too, in supporting this part of our journey.

The treatment process involved genetic counselling, fertility counselling, and more tests and appointments. I remember sitting in labs waiting for bloods to be taken and then waiting for appointments in the mail. In fact it seemed like endless waiting, thinking of all the many people faced with illness who live like this just to stay well or even alive. We were doing this simply for a chance of realising our dream of becoming parents. How privileged we were.

My response to the IVF stimulation was incredible; something I am still proud of. My now forty-one-year-old body produced fourteen eggs in one month. The high amount needed provided more options for the genetic hurdles we were facing. I still remember the delight of seeing all the follicles developing inside me on the ultrasound screen! I felt the closest I imagine it feels to being pregnant, physically and emotionally. I remember walking around the park (hard to believe I had run marathons prior to this as it now took all my energy to get through the day) feeling the pressure of the developing follicles and incredible protectiveness over them. I was nervously excited about all it potentially meant for us.

I remember standing in church feeling this growing response; really feeling I could praise God from that previously big gap inside me. God had heard me. At the same time though, I was being challenged in my mind about whether I would still praise Him as much if it was not successful?

I made a decision that, yes, I would praise Him. I strongly believed it was possible to live happy, fulfilled lives without children. But I didn't want us to be the ones to prove it.

Egg collection time was one of the most wonderful days for me. The feeling of euphoria was wonderful, though perhaps enhanced by the light sedative and opioid dose! I remember sitting in the lovely big recovery La-Z-Boy afterwards, sharing tea and toast with my husband, watching little birds come and go in the huge treetops with the sun filtering through. It was one of my favourite scenes, and we were feeling so very happy. We really enjoyed that moment. The staff at the fertility clinic were the best. They equipped us with all the information for us to make decisions, and so caringly and professionally guided us through every step of the process.

Instead of going home to rest I decided I wanted to visit my favourite shopping mall to celebrate at a café. My precious eggs were safe! We had a nice time and purchased a beautiful Israeli handcrafted scented candle with rose petals interwoven in the wax. We decided it would be lit to celebrate the hoped-for IVF success – and with fourteen harvested eggs this was looking very likely.

In a day or so we received a phone call from the embryologist to say four eggs had naturally fertilised, but one was looking immature. We were stunned: fourteen eggs and only four embryos? But still we consoled ourselves that it only required one for a baby and we hung on in hope. The next phone call from the embryologist was to inform us that, sadly, the remaining three embryos had fragmented as they divided--a sign that genetically things were not well. After such high hopes there were no embryos suitable for transfer. Those three little embryos were the closest my husband and I ever came to becoming parents. It was strange because even at that stage I loved them.

The feeling of loss was immeasurable. We quietly lit our precious candle in our little home and watched its beauty as it burned. We prayed and cried and supported each other closely. One of our dear single friends came around with flowers and hugged my tear-covered face; it meant so much to me. Our pastor came and just sat and prayed with us. My husband found this especially comforting. Friends brought soup and flowers and sent messages of support. The e-mail support of a friend who had been through a similar journey helped us greatly.

A couple of weeks later, to ease the pain, we flew to see my husband's parents and took time to break up the journey of grief. The pain of lost hope was deep, but the beauty of having now shared our journey openly with our friends and families made it a far easier grief to carry.

The reality of having closure to this part of the journey was so helpful. No longer did I have to wonder, "Could I be pregnant?" We could make plans for the future; a future without children of our own in it. I feel so privileged to have experienced this journey, to have sat in fertility waiting rooms sharing this unique journey of infertility without speaking a word with those who also sat and waited.

We had realised that on going into the IVF treatment we would risk losing the contentment we had finally gained in our infertility journey up until then, and knew we would not be able to simply pick it up where we had left off. Slowly we began to heal, and indeed, we were able to praise God within the reality of infertility.

As I write I have just turned forty-three. We celebrated by driving to a mountain village and staying in a hotel my husband had booked that looked out to the mountains reflecting the light of a full moon. In the morning we sipped tea on the balcony as the sun came up, reflecting on the mountain peaks above us.

Making the most of the incredibly clear sunny weather, we later took a flight in a small ski plane, landing on two of the glaciers before circling the mountain. We gasped at the greatness of creation then drove back home filled with more wonderful memories of living life in all its fullness.

We are proving that it is possible to live very happy and fulfilled lives with purpose without having children, even when they are so greatly longed for. My prayer of always wanting children to be part of our lives continues to be answered many times over, especially through our many nephews, nieces, and two very special goddaughters. The gift of international child sponsorship and related projects has greater significance now. It provides a chance to help parents that yearn to give their children the basics of life.

We have a great group of friends. Many are younger than us and many are single. We like to go on adventures with them. Adventures involving the outdoors and great cafes, something that being childfree tends to make room for. To simply pack up and go travelling with minimal planning needed is great. A little three-man tent has lent itself to some amazing memories with the promise of many more to come.

One key for me in not being career-oriented is realising it is okay to work part-time, staying freed up to enjoy running, making home a nice place to be, and spending time doing "kiddie things" with my friends and their children.

A lot has to do with celebrating what we do have--each other and many choices, rather than spending too much time being sad about what we don't have. Indeed the gap of infertility is never filled. Other things just become a lot bigger, so the gap has less room. And some of these other things are wonderful.

Forever infertility is part of our story, and I can honestly say I wouldn't change our story for anything.

DESTINED, CREATED FOR ME

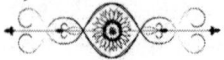

Ellen's Story

I was nineteen when I learned I wouldn't be able to have children. After experiencing pain through much of my teens, I was eventually put to sleep for a thorough examination. The doctors discovered a leaking appendix had been infecting my fallopian tubes for many years, clubbing and flattening them. They also removed a large benign cyst on one of my ovaries.

I clearly remember my doctor telling me the prognosis. A dear family friend, he felt terrible they hadn't caught the problem years before and waited until after my high school graduation to break the news to me. Naturally I was quite upset until my pastor asked me, "Do you want to have children right now?" When I told him no he responded, "Then don't worry about it until you have to." It was good advice and I took it.

Before my husband and I got engaged, I told him I couldn't have children. Tom's mother and father had six children in less than six years and Tom wanted a large family too. Recently I asked him why he had married me when he knew I couldn't give him children. He said, "I liked you. I knew God would take care of it." A typical "Tom" answer.

As newly married virgins, sex in that first year was exciting— learning to give and take, to love and be loved, to trust each other with our secret desires. And we were so hopeful. Even though the doctors had said there was absolutely no way I could ever get pregnant, we knew God delights in impossibilities. In the bible, hadn't Sarah, Rachel, Hannah, and Elizabeth heard the same words? And look what happened to them—they all got pregnant! We knew it took only one little sperm to get through that flat tube to make a baby. God could do that easily!

A year went by. Of course we never used any kind of birth control, ever. Every woman who's had trouble getting pregnant knows the monthly cycle: sex, sex, sex. A day late. Two days late. Three. Four. Hope is high, hope is deliriously joyful. Then the inevitable, hateful flow of blood, tears, numbness, depression. I remember it bothered me more than it bothered Tom. He's always been a patient soul.

Year two. Tom was appointed to pastor a small church in southwest Texas near the Mexican border. I wrote to my doctor asking if anything could be done–was there some procedure that would repair my tubes? He recommended a local specialist. If anyone could help me it would be this man.

We consulted with our new specialist and after a laparoscopy he told us he could reconstruct my fallopian tubes. We were ecstatic and scheduled the surgery. I remember waking up from the anesthetic to see a woman sitting on the side of my bed. Smiling up at her, I waited for her to tell me I could now get pregnant. Instead she used words like "too much damage," "inoperable," and "impossible."

I looked across the room to the empty bed on my right. Just the day before a young woman in her twenties had lain there telling me she was having an abortion because she and her husband simply didn't want a second child. She had her "procedure" and left the hospital. Wait a minute, God, are you paying attention here? Did you mean to rub my face in it like this?

This was the first time I saw Tom's faith falter. We were so sure the surgery was our answer. We truly believed we would be "normal" after I woke up. When we left the hospital we went straight to a nearby camping area where we stayed for a couple of nights, walking and walking and walking and crying out to God. But life doesn't afford many days to indulge in walking and crying; life moves on and we must move with it. Tom reminded me that he didn't marry me to have babies, it wasn't just "Ellen's problem," and together we would get through the pain and find the joy.

Year three. In between "impossible" and "too much damage," I had heard the woman say, "You're a good candidate for in vitro fertilization." I grabbed those words and didn't let go. At that time IVF cost about $4,000USD per cycle—a lot of money in 1985. We didn't have it, but we were thankful my uncle did and was willing to help us out. We arranged to stay for two weeks with my brother-in-law, close to the hospital where I would go for daily injections and ultrasounds. Our specialist assured us his team had a high success rate. All I had to do was call when my period started and he would get the ball rolling. We were sure to have a baby within the year.

We made the arrangements and waited for my period to start. And then waited some more… and then some more. Hope killed in that hospital room began to live again. Of course this was how God worked! How like Him to wait until we were about to do it ourselves, for Him to show His sovereignty. I woke every morning almost literally holding my breath. Throughout the day I would imagine how I would tell my family, how they would react. Tom was more cautious – he learns a lot faster than I do. Tom and I agreed that on day sixty, if I hadn't started my period, we would go to the clinic and get a pregnancy test.

Day sixty arrived. We went to the clinic and I gave the sample. Forty-five minutes later we heard the doctor say we had a "weak positive." I was pregnant! The joy was indescribable; the gratitude to God unquenchable. We went to the grocery store and bought two big T-bone steaks to grill and celebrate. Between the store and home I felt the bubble burst; I felt the familiar devastation of my body betraying me. I felt the familiar dreaded flow.

Tom's reaction to these times was to trust God more and cling to Him more tightly. My reaction was to give in to anger, hatred, and jealousy. I had so many questions God would not or, in my estimation, could not answer for me. "God, you parted the Red Sea. You raised people from the dead. You made the blind man see. I'm asking you to send one – ONE egg down a flat fallopian tube. You CAN do it. You just WON'T. And you say you love me?" I was asking God to move a finger and He wouldn't do it.

I began to hate sex. There didn't seem to be any point to it. I could never think, "Maybe it happened this time – maybe we just made a baby." I knew it was hopeless. Sex became something I did to keep my husband happy. After all, why drive a car for miles and miles and miles and miles – endlessly – all the while knowing you're never going to get where you want to go? That's how sex felt to me. I wish I could have kept that feeling from Tom, but hatred is a very difficult emotion to hide. Infertility isn't a pretty thing; before it produces a good marriage it can send a couple to hell and back. Our sex life went round and round in an endless cycle of desire and rejection (Tom), anger and guilt (me), and enough sadness for both of us.

I began to feel like damaged goods. I felt guilty Tom was stuck with me – it was completely my fault we couldn't have children. I hated my body – hated the way it was irregular with my periods and fooled us so many times into hoping and wishing, only to throw us down in disappointment time after time after time. I hated the parts that gave me pain and would never produce a child – would never fulfill what they were designed for. To me, having fallopian tubes that never allowed an egg to reach the uterus was similar to having legs that don't function or kidneys that don't work. They're a useless part of the body, broken and damaged beyond repair.

Not only my marital relationship suffered, I continued to struggle with God. How could He treat me this way? How would it hurt Him to, at the very least, just make my periods regular? How could He be so cruel – to make me late month after month, year after year, and then dash me against the rocks just when I managed to pull myself up one more time to believe in miracles? I felt like I was Charlie Brown and God was Lucy holding the football. "C'mon, Ellen! I won't do it again, I promise! This time I'll hold it in place – really!" How could I be stupid enough to believe God cared?

I wondered if He thought I wouldn't be a good mother. Could that be the reason He wouldn't let me get pregnant? I saw so many teenage girls getting pregnant and figured He thought they were better than me. I felt God had judged me and pronounced His sentence: unworthy.

We picked ourselves up and looked once again to IVF. In November 1985 when my period began at the right time, I called the clinic to tell them we would be able to start the next day. The woman on the phone said, "Yes, you're in the GIFT (gamete intra-fallopian transfer) program, correct?" GIFT, a procedure our specialist developed, requires a woman to have open tubes which I, of course, did not have.

I assured her that no, I was in the IVF program and needed to make an appointment to start my procedure. Again she questioned, "Are you sure you're not in the GIFT program?" Then she said, "Why don't you come in the day after tomorrow, have your first ultrasound and injection, and the doctor will talk to you."

Tom and I went to our specialist the next day and camped outside his office until he came back from his rounds. We insisted on seeing him right away. He took us in, closed the door, sat us down, and informed us he was no longer running the IVF program. He was only doing GIFT procedures now and besides, they'd never had a successful pregnancy with IVF.

Numbness and devastation set in. Once again so close, just to have the door slammed in our faces. How could I believe in a loving God when everything inside me was screaming, "Why,

God, why? How could you do this to me?" Once again Tom was the rock, the one who knew God had a plan of His own.

We went home, fought once in a while, made up every time, lived life, tried to forget, moved on. We became reconciled to the fact that pregnancy was never going to happen.

Five months later in April 1986 we attended a dinner at our church. The speaker was the director of a crisis center in a small neighboring town. As she spoke she ran down a list of the people they were currently housing. When she mentioned a woman giving up her baby for adoption, I heard bells ringing in my head. The words went through my mind, "That's your baby." The closing twenty minutes of the meeting were the longest of my life...

When the meeting ended I approached her and asked if the woman adopting out was going through an agency. Apparently she had yet to decide. I wrote my phone number down and as I handed it to the woman I said, "Would you please ask her if I could have her baby?" Less than twenty-four hours later the woman called to tell us, "She said yes!"

We immediately contacted a lawyer friend who contacted the birth mother's doctor. This wasn't the first time we'd considered adoption. We'd had several calls through the years asking if we were interested in a "friend of a friend's daughter's baby" – all fell through. Once we were even offered twins! At the time private adoptions were still legal in Texas and generally much less expensive than agency adoptions.

Of course the time of waiting was like dancing on the edge of a cliff. So thankful, so joyous, yet knowing that one small misstep could end it all. But the birthmother never wavered, even when we insisted on a closed adoption in which information is sealed and identities are kept private.

The doctors did an ultrasound and said the baby would be born in mid-August. The birthmother insisted the baby would be born in July. On July 9 I flew from Texas to Wisconsin to visit my mother; the next morning Tom called to tell me we had a son.

A day later Tom and I held thirty-hour-old Daniel Evan in our arms. We took him home and surprised our church family during the sermon on Sunday morning. After so many disappointments we'd told only two people about the adoption; I'll never forget the tears and celebration during that service.

I still don't know why God allows circumstances to develop that give His children hope leading seemingly nowhere. Sometimes I'm still sad I'll never be pregnant, never feel life grow in my body, never feel the wonder of a baby moving. I'll never know what it would be like to see the look in Tom's eyes if I could tell him I was pregnant and we were going to have a baby.

But I know Daniel was chosen for us, just as surely as I know God never left us nor forsook us through it all. I know that before the foundation of the world God knew Daniel would need a mom and a dad and we would be the ones for him. The moment he was placed in my arms, the anger, the hatred of infertility was suddenly…gone. After all, if I could have gotten pregnant, I wouldn't be holding my Daniel in my arms. I knew in that moment I wouldn't trade this child for a hundred of "my own" biological children. Such is the healing miracle of a child given by God to be mine just as surely as if He'd grown in my womb.

Tom never got his large family. Daniel is our only child. Sometimes I ask God about that, wondering why He didn't give us more children. But I've changed over the years. I no longer react in anger when my questions go unanswered. I've joined Tom's side – knowing that what God is asking for, longing for, is my trust. Trust that believes in His love and care for me, no matter what circumstances surround me. The most precious gift I can give Him is this trust, knowing nothing comes to me He doesn't allow, for my good and my blessing—and His glory. We ask our children to trust us this way; how can we expect God to desire anything less from His beloved children?

LOSS, LIFE AND LOVE

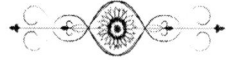

Priscilla's Story

THIS is our story, the story of four babies who once were and now will be only known in the certainty of Heaven.

Our story begins after five years of marriage, when we returned home from living overseas to settle and start our family. We bought our first home with large rooms to fill and large dreams to match. We never anticipated any problems, why would we? One may've thought I would have known better, having worked in a Neonatal Intensive Care Unit for the past six years. I had come across varying degrees of fertility problems, so it wasn't news to me that some women struggle to have their "blessing" fulfilled.

It's an exciting prospect when a couple decides to begin the baby adventure. You dream of healthy, chubby, happy babies. They may look like you, have your husband's eyes, or worse, your temper, and so the dreams go on. For many of us the dream begins at the birth, but for many others of us, the dream can be crushed at your first or second scan.

This was how it was for Glenn and me. I got pregnant relatively quickly and so the excitement began. Psalm 139 was spoken out in faith and my every waking hour was highlighted with this baby's existence. By the time I was six weeks pregnant, two sets of booties had been produced and the third was well on its way to completion. To say my parents were excited would have been a gross understatement. Rugby balls had been purchased and window shopping in the baby stores commenced. Unlike some who don't share their news until the magical twelve week mark, our joy was quickly shared with many.

After talking with my midwife, we decided to get a scan at fourteen weeks to confirm our dates. We were more than confident in our baby's well-being and my morning sickness had disappeared at about eight weeks. I remember saying, "I feel so well, I don't even feel pregnant." How those words would haunt me!

We arrived for the scan with huge expectation. I got on the table, eagerly awaiting our first glimpse of the one who would fill the booties so lovingly made, the one who would kick the ball my dad had bought, even wondering at the chance of twins.

Surely there just can't be an easy way to tell expectant parents bad news. The lady who scanned us was quiet, too quiet. I knew something was wrong when she asked how many weeks we thought the baby was. When I said fourteen weeks, our dreams were shattered in one foul swoop. The baby had no heartbeat and looked about eight or nine weeks' gestation. Our joy of pregnancy was lost that day. Never again would it hold the same innocent excitement it had that first time.

Oh how we grieved; the failure I felt as a woman and a wife was incredible. To be told miscarriage was common brought no comfort at all. I had lost our big, healthy, happy baby, the one who would look like me, have his father's eyes, my sanguine personality. That's the baby I grieved for.

We got a silver ring for my little finger and engraved it with "in memory of our first." I found it hard to grieve when there was no funeral, no body as such. It was as though scan pictures were our baby's only memorial. Everywhere I looked I saw babies and pregnant women. My mind felt assaulted at every turn.

Returning to church was difficult. Returning to my relationship with God even more so. When I tried to pray, all I did was cry, so much so that in one journal entry, I wrote of my fear that I was going crazy. Standing in church, I felt like a fraud. I was a leader, one meant to encourage those in distress, telling them that God was faithful and true even in the hard times.

Yet here I was angry and disappointed and discouraged in my own time of trial. I felt offended when the worship leader spoke of our ever-faithful God, one who can do the impossible.

I knew I was in a bad space and in desperate need of connection with the One I felt so disconnected from. I then heard a story of a pastor who, when praising God for saving his young son after being found facedown in a pool, felt challenged by God.

The man related how God spoke to him, asking if he would still praise His name even if his son had died? Would God be any less real if the pastors son hadn't survived? Was his motivation for praising God based on the truth of God or was it based on his son being saved?

I realized that God was still God, even in my disappointment and grief; my loss hadn't changed the truth about who God was.

Time passed and we felt ready to forge ahead again. We were full of faith that God would deliver His promise. I fell pregnant four months later. Somewhat bruised, I again proclaimed Psalm 139. Surely we wouldn't miscarry a second time! But I didn't tell the world just in case…

We went for a scan at six weeks and saw the heartbeat, which I heard means there is a very good chance the pregnancy will progress successfully. The relief was tangible. We were on our way.

We went for another scan around three months. I'd had a little bit of spotting but no pain or cramps, and some morning sickness. No longer was I dreaming there might be twins, just a heartbeat.

I couldn't believe it – our baby had died at nine weeks. I shut God down this time. I had believed for this baby. I felt that I had allowed myself to dream again. What was the point in His promises if they didn't come to pass? I was angry and bitter. I felt like a failure. My useless body couldn't maintain a pregnancy.

November 1, 2001
(journal extract)

Yesterday we lost our second baby. I don't understand. What's the point in praying for protection when protection doesn't come? I understand one baby, but why two? People want to pray for us, to fight against the plans of the devil, but God is bigger than that... "Greater is he who is in us, than he who is in the world." Why is this happening to us, why do people who don't give a hoot about God and do bad things get babies and we, who love God and would be good parents, lose two babies? I have been pregnant twice and have nothing to show for it! Off for another dreaded D&C!

As I hadn't told the world of our pregnancy, no one really knew what was happening to us. To be honest, I wished I had. People not acknowledging our loss was far more painful than dealing with their comments. It felt as though our baby hadn't existed. This time I asked to bring our baby home. Its tiny white container was absurd but strangely comforting. The staff had kindly attached a purple flower. As we buried our baby under an olive tree, my husband prayed and my heart broke; it was so painful to bury that little white box.

Here we were again, back in the reruns of grief. I was disillusioned and feeling the distance in my relationship with God. I stopped talking to Him, but thankfully my friends didn't. They prayed while I just cried and slowly I came back to Him and I felt us cry together. The thought of God grieving with me helped me open up to Him again. I still didn't understand why He hadn't prevented this loss, but I now knew He cared.

* * *

January 7, 2002

Well today we found out I am pregnant again. Thank you, Lord, for our third blessing. We prayed this morning that this will be a healthy, full-term baby.

This time we went through the local hospital's recurrent miscarriage clinic. I had blood taken twice a week to check my HCG levels and weekly scans from six to fourteen weeks. I attended a relaxation class, stopped work, and was told not to clean, go out anywhere, (including church), for the first twelve weeks of this pregnancy. I was on partial bed rest and my parents moved in to support us. It's not so strict now but then the instructions were NO STRESS!

On February 16, my husband's birthday, I awoke around midnight and was losing huge amounts of blood. I remember screaming. I was absolutely distraught and disappointed beyond belief. We made an appointment with the recurrent miscarriage clinic for February 19. The nurse told me to stay on complete bed rest and watch the bleeding, saying my last blood results were excellent and it wasn't necessarily bad news. It was an awful two days wavering between faith and disbelief that it seemed to be happening again.

Well Lord, I sit here the night before the scan that will check again on the well-being of our baby. I admit I'm so scared of our baby being dead, but I have to remember that faith is something you have even and especially when it's unseen. Lord, give me the strength to cope, whatever the result. This is so hard, but God, I still thank you for all I have...an incredible family, an incredible husband, and great friends. Bless my parents for their commitment to me. Please, Lord, stop this bleeding, continue to protect our baby, continue to let him/her grow strong and healthy IN JESUS NAME!

The scan showed the baby was still alive but if a large area of bleeding outside the sac wasn't absorbed it could cause a miscarriage at twenty-one weeks or so. Friends and family prayed on our behalf. I was so frightened. The stress was unbearable. But thankfully the following week's scan showed the clot had been so totally absorbed they couldn't find it. On September 14, 2002 I gave birth to a healthy, strong, full-term baby girl we named Georgia Zoe.

I went on to have a further two losses between Georgia and our second live baby we named Harper Sue. Although it was still painful, once I had Georgia, miscarrying was not as difficult. I could get pregnant relatively easily, so I just needed to keep going until a pregnancy continued successfully.

I would love to say how I stood in faith, how my relationship with God was strengthened, but it wouldn't be true. Many occasions were rocky, but my incredible family and friends stood in the gap and prayed on my behalf when I felt unable to.

Fourteen months after Harper's birth, we had a premature baby boy we named Finn Jeremy at thirty-two weeks after my membranes ruptured at twenty-eight weeks. Here we ended our fertility issues and called it quits. We were emotionally drained from what seemed an eternity of waiting for my period to be late, checking for signs of bleeding every time I went to the bathroom when I was pregnant, wanting to feel morning sickness, and being frightened when I didn't. The scans, the blood tests, the lost spontaneity in our love life! It was a harrowing presence in our marriage. We were ready to call it a day. I was tired of responding to the altar call in tears. I was ready to feel normal again.

We have been richly blessed with our three children but still acknowledge those we lost. We made it through this time of fertility problems, and our relationship is the richer for it. It could have gone either way--brought us closer together or pushed us apart. It was incredibly tiring and emotional for all involved; the support of our family, particularly my parents, friends, and church through these six long years was invaluable. I thank God for making the unbearable bearable.

FAITH AND PERSEVERANCE

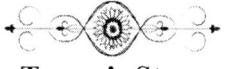

Teresa's Story

"THERE are three things that are never satisfied, four that never say, 'Enough!: the grave, the barren womb, land which is never satisfied with water, and fire which never says, 'Enough!' Proverbs 30:15-16, NIV

Encountering Grief

"Your Word says you are pure, just, and holy, God. I don't feel this right now, and I know my heart must choose to believe it. I am angry that I can't get pregnant. I feel worn down and sick of this roller coaster. I am feeling like this is a cruel joke from you. I know you are the giver of good things and Satan is the deceiver... but all of this doesn't make sense to me..." -- Journal Entry

I arrived home to find my husband laying in bed reading. He saw from the look on my face that something was terribly wrong. Tears filled my eyes and my knees weakened as I collapsed on the floor in a heap of despair.

A dear friend who was living overseas had come home for the weekend to have a baby shower in Michigan and shop for baby supplies with her mother and me. My response to seeing her blossoming pregnancy took me by surprise. That night I sobbed for hours, gripped by the fear of never having a belly growing with life and a baby shower of my own.

Jason and I had been trying to conceive for a year. Fear had been lurking nearby, but when it reared its ugly head that day it took on a whole new form and intensity. Since then fear has threatened to creep its way back into my mind and paralyze me. I must always be on guard against that thief of joy.

A few close friends have travelled the road of infertility; some waiting a few years for their children, others still waiting ten years after their journey began. My heart ached for them. As I found myself in this place of frustration and disappointment, that ache reached a new level of understanding, more familiar than I would have liked.

This strong desire for children has always been a part of me. It resides deep within, as though stitched into the fabric of my being. I believed then that God would use this desire for His glory, and still do most days. Perhaps He is just choosing to use it in a vastly different fashion than I had in mind, for "My thoughts are not your thoughts, neither are your ways my ways, declares the LORD" (Isaiah 55:8-9, NIV).

God's dreams for my life may be quite different from mine, or possibly my dreams are just taking longer to come true than I'd hoped. Often we approach life with an expectation of what God's will should be and assume He will help us fulfill that. We're then presented with a choice as to what we'll do when life does not work out as we'd expected. While learning to accept my situation as God's will, I have to focus on a twenty-four-hour period when struggling to keep going during the most difficult times. God sets the stage and I'm striving to learn my part.

Grief became known to me when my desire to conceive was not forthcoming. Faith and grace have kept me afloat on a daily basis as I learn to cohabit with the pain. At a young age I chose to make God the Lord of my life. He still holds this position, even when my dreams appear shattered and grief has seemingly taken over the corner they held in my heart.

I've often felt confused about why God has allowed me to walk this path. I've seen Him bless my life, felt Him carry me, and known Him to answer prayers. I struggle to understand these feelings of abandonment by the One who said, "I will never leave you nor forsake you." Will the rest of my life be less than desirable? Will it lack joy and happiness? Is this desire to be used simply for my career as a registered nurse (RN), caring for patients and families at the hospital, especially children and newborns?

At times I question how this trial could be beneficial to my life. Will our marriage survive its crushing pressure? My mind reels with questions and frustration, then peace overcomes me. I want to know how to keep this peace. I long to grasp how I am led to peaceful waters even when my heart is breaking.

Encountering true grief on a roller coaster of twists, turns, ups and downs presents critical choices. I have had to decide how to banish this grief to the sidelines of my life, rather than let it be a constant power yelling for my attention. Most importantly, I long to know where it will take my relationship with God as He walks this life with me.

Wise Choices

"Faith never knows where it is being led, but it knows and loves the One who is leading." – Oswald Chambers

Several years as an RN in a neonatal intensive care unit (NICU) has helped shape a lot of my views on infertility treatments. I've seen litters of babies born: multiples of three, four, and more in greatly varying conditions. Some have minimal or no limitations; others have severe physical and mental delays. The parents' heartache and the pain these little ones endure during their long NICU stay is gut wrenching. And this is only the beginning of raising these children. I have become acutely aware of the potential drawbacks of taking fertility medication and the risks that could be involved, even with monitoring and direction by a skilled physician.

I have been determined not to compromise my faith, my future, and God's plan for my life. I never want to force my agenda, because I know God's love for me is pure and His plan for my life, no matter what I am struggling with, is so much better than my own plans (Jeremiah 29:11). Scripture tells us, "But my people did not listen to my voice... So I gave them over to their stubborn hearts to follow their own devices" (Psalm 81:11-12, NIV). Those who followed their own counsel and trusted their own hearts suffered further heartache, pain, and even death.

God's heart is more trustworthy than mine. I want Him to be the one to direct my path, no matter where it leads, because I cannot always see the destination. He does. I do believe in medical advancements and know they can be a blessing. But I also believe if we ask Him, God grants us the wisdom to use these wisely.

Out of Reach

"I know you must have a good plan for our family, but I don't feel like you do right now. Fear has come again and the peace I had last month seems out of reach....." --Journal Entry

It was spring when my husband graduated from his Masters degree program, landed a job, and we started trying for a family. The timing seemed perfect. I could be a stay-at-home mom and put my energy into growing godly children. After a few months of trying, my doctor recommended we undergo some blood tests to make sure there were no obvious problems. There were no issues with the test results.

We knew it can sometimes take up to a year to conceive, and we'd been under stress with jobs and house building. We had conceived and miscarried a year into our marriage, so we felt sure we would soon be pregnant again. Toward Christmas my doctor recommended Clomid. Jason and I felt strongly about that drug and the lack of proper monitoring we had observed, so we declined. We decided to try naturally for a year and continue asking God to bless us. If nothing happened we would seek further advice.

And so, after fourteen months of trying, we decided to pay our doctor another visit. Due to the irregularity of days between my menstrual cycles, my doctor wondered if I may not be ovulating properly. Again she suggested Clomid. This time she offered me an ultrasound after each cycle and prior to intercourse to check whether too many mature follicles were forming and increasing the risk of a pregnancy of multiples. As this sounded like a viable option, we agreed. If at any time we were uncomfortable with a procedure, we could discontinue.

Over the following four months we entered the world of Clomid, ultrasounds, injections, and timed intercourse. The medical procedures went well; the outcome did not. No pregnancy. With each procedure our hope soared, only to be followed by disappointment. My doctor could see the heartache setting in and recommended we visit an infertility specialist. We took a few months off to regain our composure and continued asking God for a miracle so we wouldn't have to take that next step.

Private Pain

"What a painful experience. I never knew! There are days of hope, anger, devastation, frustration, and God's mercy. You have given us so much grace, God, to help us go on and to stay positive. Please don't let these emotions make my decisions or affect my outlook on life. May you rain down grace on me and remind me of truth. Please bless us with a baby this month!" --Journal Entry

Questions about when we would be expanding our family became more frequent as my husband's school days drifted further behind us. When we reached the point of seeking medical advice, we decided it was time to tell our friends and family about our situation and ask them to pray for us. We made it clear that our medical details were private but we were open to discussing how we were emotionally. Since then I've had moments when I am able to feel these prayers carrying me. They have helped to lift the black cloud from over my head, and wipe the tears from my eyes. This hope and peace is evidence in itself that God is walking this journey with me, and answering prayers on my behalf.

Keeping my marriage sacred, as well as showing my husband honor and respect, are vital to me. This journey is painful for him too, and I mustn't forget we are a team walking this road together. Even though he expresses himself in different ways or aches at different times, it's a daily surrender for him, knowing he cannot ease the ache in his wife's heart. At times he has wondered if there must be something wrong with him they haven't detected. I want to help him by being the best wife I can be. If I choose to talk about this topic, I also need to think of what will be resonating in his ears and heart.

God did not intend for us to walk alone, but to live in community with one another. "Carry each other's burdens, and in this way you will fulfill the law of Christ" (Galatians 6:2, NIV). It has been important to me to be real and transparent with my friends and family (with discretion). Romans 12:15 (NIV) tells us to "Rejoice with those who rejoice; mourn with those who mourn." The words of encouragement from friends and family I've kept since the beginning of this journey continue to bless and carry me. Email updates on where we're at and what God is teaching us allow people to pray for us and gives me opportunities to praise Him for His goodness. I delight in knowing I'm learning through this pain and that others can too. It gives me hope to know some good may come out of it.

Surrender

"God, this is painful. My heart aches so deep I can barely breathe. You tell me you will never leave me nor forsake me. I will cling to that. You say you love me and I will watch for your love." --Journal Entry

After a year of trying, grief started setting in like a fierce storm making its way to shore. While I was jogging one morning listening to music, God spoke to me about surrendering. He impressed upon me that what He can do in my life is so much greater than those dreams I clutch on to. Yet I wondered how I could possibly give up this desire to have children. I was unsure how I could get rid of this ache in my gut, so bad some days it seemed someone was literally tearing out my insides. If I did surrender, would He remove this pain? That would be a glorious thing, but I was unsure of the direction my life would then take. It seemed scary: so many questions, not many answers. The one clear thing was He wanted me to surrender my dreams to Him.

I felt upset that seeking God's will and accepting each turn had led me to what I felt was a dead end. I wasn't prepared for the fact that having chosen God's way in my life, I would still have major trials, rather than blessing beyond measure. I was surprised that choosing to follow Him did not protect me from the pain and disappointment that were becoming a familiar way of life. The Bible says in John 16:33 (NIV) "… In this world you will have trouble. But take heart! I have overcome the world." I was at a crossroad, questioning if this God I had chosen to follow really was who He said He was. I had to decide whether or not to keep following and trusting Him when it felt like He had abandoned me. If God could not help me, who would?

I now know I was mourning a loss; grieving for an unfulfilled dream. The pain I felt as my fingers were pried away from the grip I had on that dream was real. Reality was separated from desire. I see death as a separation between the soul and the body. When Christ died there was a brief separation from the Father, the darkest time in history. We can choose to be separated from God or live in eternity with Him when our physical bodies die. God's desires the latter. We are not made for separation. I see separation from our dreams as similar to a death.

I threw myself into the Bible and gained strength from God's truth. Peace would come over me as I read, yet when I closed the page I struggled to hold onto it. I knew I was going to have to be constantly in God's Word to keep the lies of the evil one far from me and maintain stability. I started studying who this God I say I serve really is. I wanted to overcome doubt and learn to trust when everything seemed to argue against it.

In those pages I found story after story of His faithfulness and never-changing nature. He was attentive to the cries of His children, not always in human timing, but in perfect timing: His timing. I looked at Noah in Genesis and the faith he had. He was told to build an ark for when the flood came. Over one hundred years passed before the rains appeared. It must've felt as though God had forgotten.

I believe Noah would have had some questions about God following through or whether he had heard God correctly. I also believe, knowing he was human, that Noah would also have had some raw thoughts toward God and yet he did not walk away. Scripture says Noah was blameless and walked faithfully with God. Could I do this too?

I began rediscovering things I'd forgotten. Truths I had known in my mind and heart now spoke to my spirit in a new way, directly to my pain and fears. I was committing to seeking God throughout this journey, a God who never changes. When the road got rough, I was going to do what was needed to stay close to my Father. He loved me and had promised to help me in this world. He sees the big picture and promises to prosper me, even when I don't understand. Jesus tells his followers in John 10:10 (NIV), "The thief comes only to steal, kill and destroy; I have come that they may have life, and have it to the full." I determined to know more of Him and hear His voice, because I knew He would lead me to greener pastures and still waters (Ps. 23:2, NIV).

High Hopes

"We finished our final round of IUI this month and this week I found out I was not pregnant. I feel a peace though, like God has a

plan and is going to answer our prayers some day with our own pregnancy. My heart feels calm and still." --Journal Entry

After two years of trying to conceive, it was time to visit the specialist. I was learning that often you don't know what you will do at the next step until you come to it. Jason had been adamant that we not discuss each option till it was necessary. This focused me on the here and now rather than worrying about things we may never encounter. I could have hope for the moment.

We decided to remain faithful to our convictions, cover all things in prayer, and seek God's plan rather than push our own desires by undertaking options we knew weren't right for us. Strong desires can sometimes take over us as women, hugely challenging the respect and submission due to our spouse. To end up with a child but lose my marriage was not the desired result.

For the next sixteen months we visited the specialists often. We attempted IUI nine times, occasionally with a month off in between. The doctors explained the procedures well and were understanding of our convictions about what we would and wouldn't undertake. We proceeded cautiously.

The timing for these procedures was exact, the trips to the offices were intense and exhausting. The perseverance, energy, interruption to normal life, and the emotion that went into the process were grueling. Only the longing to come out with a healthy pregnancy kept us going. This was absolutely our greatest roller coaster ride as a couple during this journey. Our hopes were high as we continued praying for healing, as well as thanking God for the medical advancements we could use. We were grateful we had the financial resources to take part in such science and for being of one heart and mind in our desires and decisions.

On our final attempt the doctor recommended we move on to IVF. I asked that he please let us try one more round with the IUI as we had found a good medication dose and were not ready to consider IVF. He agreed. My husband and I knew we were physically and mentally nearing exhaustion. With each month that came, our hope would rise, no matter how hard we tried to restrain it.

One warm, sunny June day in 2010, I headed to the doctor's office for my last round of IUI. I felt sad and scared, yet I sensed a glimmer of hope way off in the corner of my heart. I pondered if this could be the time or if my heart would be let down once again. Emotion took over and I cried all the way to the office and all the way home.

Dwelling Places

"God, if you can satisfy me and you do meet all my needs, why is this longing in my heart so strong to have children? Please destroy this desire within me if you won't allow me to have children.....I want to live victoriously, but feel devoured with pain and despair..." --- Journal Entry

There's a battle within my soul to believe God has not forgotten me but is weaving something beautiful out of this big picture. Among the many emotional ups and downs, fear tends to go the first round, then once that is taken off the court, anger is right there, ready for a match. When I can say no to fear I go into fighting mode. I think, "I can fight this battle, I'm going to come out on top. God is going to help me do this and answer my prayers!" That power can be fleeting. On days when I am weary and wonder if victory will ever come or if the battle is going to destroy me, anger wells up – mostly toward God.

Psalm 100:4, (NIV) tells me to, "Enter his gates with thanksgiving and his courts with praise; give thanks to him and praise his name." This is the last thing I want to do when my heart is angry. If I view God as a lightning-throwing monster, aiming at humans below, my frustration turns toward Him. But if I view Him in light of who He has proven himself to be over thousands of years, I see Him working from outside my circumstances, calling out to me through my weakness and limitations. The very thing causing my pain can be redeemed and become an instrument of grace. When I've chosen to let anger dwell in my life, I quit thanking God for the many blessings He has given me. This in turn draws me away from the closeness of God Himself or even the interaction of people that could bring comfort.

"Whoever dwells in the shelter of the Most High will rest in the shadow of the Almighty" (Psalm 91:1, NIV). While studying this topic of "resting in the shadow of the Almighty," suddenly the reality of it flooded my mind. I could see God standing like a tall oak tree in the middle of a grassy field. Next to that tree I receive shade and protection from sun, wind, rain, and other dangers. I'm near my God, even able to touch Him and lean on Him when I'm weary. I can have a relationship with God and others in that shelter. I can see the beauty of God during different seasons of life. His arm reaches farther than mine and filters any harm that may be headed in my direction. I rest in peace. The closer I dwell to God, getting to know Him during the easy times of life, the easier it'll be to dwell there during the hard times, because I've learned to trust Him for who He is.

On days I choose to hold back and not have a thankful heart, I leave the security of dwelling under that mighty oak. My aches and pains of desiring a child are tugging and pulling. God is inviting me to rest in His shelter. I feel the pull and I know I have committed to follow and accept His calling to me.

Friends In Need

"Please strengthen me, Lord, as our hearts ache for children and we grow weary with impatience. Help me to live a life for you, instead of feeling dead inside and depressed by the heartaches of this current life.....Help me to see with your eyes and see life from your point of view" --Journal Entry

In the fall of 2009, two and a half years into this journey, I started feeling very depressed. I'd felt trapped before but now it became overwhelming. Feelings of hopelessness, of not wanting to live if it meant I would continue carrying this heartache of wanting children, gripped my heart like never before. I slowly came to the realization that I'd put this dream on a higher pedestal than the one I had God on.

Over the years there have been times I didn't want to talk about God's love and power in this situation because I didn't want people to think we were doing fine and then forget to pray for us or understand how difficult it is. When we're in pain we want to be understood. To hear someone say, "That must be really hard, I am so sorry," is priceless. Life becomes less lonely when others offer sympathy. The moments when friends and family stood with us in understanding gave me strength to keep going when I thought I could not.

I didn't want to spend more time wishing for tomorrow than enjoying the blessings of today. I didn't like nor want the darkness and longed to bask in God's peace once again. The power this darkness held in my life was unacceptable – particularly how it affected my marriage. I treasured my marriage and wanted to protect it and to enjoy life along the way to achieving our dream(s).

When I confessed to a dear friend that my life without having children was equal to life not worth living, I was embarrassed to be feeling this way. I didn't want to feel so hopeless and filled with anguish. I realized that somewhere over the past months I had moved out from under God's shadow. It was not a daily deliberate choice, but a gradual move motivated by pain. She helped me find the strength to face one day at a time as I waited. She reminded me that God has promised me a future with hope and this time will also prepare me for great things in my life. Good, trusted, wise friends are invaluable.

Useable Pottery

"God, I thank you for my weaknesses and for this trial. Thank you for this painful trial of waiting for children. You have protected and taught us. My acknowledgement of weakness in my life crumbles down my walls of pride, and softens my heart to people around me." --Journal Entry

I have a hope that God is doing something beautiful with this pain in my life right now. In some moments on this twisting path I have cried out to God from the pit of my stomach to take this trial away. In other moments I have thanked Him for allowing me to walk this road. There have been opportunities to learn, grow, love my husband more, mature my thinking based on God's truths, and learn about areas of pain I'd never known. I do wish it would end soon but can honestly say I'm thankful.

Hope has continued to pop up. At times I can grasp it, other times I struggle. I have come to realize hope cannot be shaken. Hope does not believe I will get what I want. Hope believes that regardless of what I have in mind, God will have the final word and His ways are higher and better than mine. Jesus is the redeeming factor in this broken world. I will put my hopes in the One who is firm and secure. When life seems to look hopeless and my future looks unclear, I will look to the One who promises to fulfill His good plan.

One thing that has kept me buoyant is being able to help others. I've chosen to try and see each day as more than an obstacle to overcome; it is alive with opportunities from the hand of God. I don't want to miss my part in these! I can regularly see God using me right where I am; I actively look for opportunities and think about ways to be thankful for where He has me right now. Following Him means bringing a touch of peace, justice, hope, and healing wherever my hands touch. My heart has been drastically changed and my ability to meet people in their pain and dis-appointment has become a reality. I now understand broken dreams, broken hearts, and broken hope. My eyes are open to the bigger reality of life in light of eternity. I'm only passing through this world where the Bible tells me I will have trials and tribu-lations.

I'd prepared to stay home with my children but since we have none as yet, I work full time as a registered nurse. Countless re-lationships have offered me opportunities to share Christ and what He's done in my life. Some of these people are walking with God or seeking to find out more about Him, simply because I was available and willing when the opportunity arose. Rather than wallowing in my sorrow, I am offering it to God and seeking ways for Him to use me today. I have been able to minister to hurting hearts because I have been there.

It's not that I have answers for others' pain. I don't even have answers for my own. I've learned that most of the time we don't need suggestions or solutions, we just want someone to sit with us and listen with a sympathetic heart. What I do have is a heart that can feel and listen and hurt with them. I hope I can be the friend to others that Job's true friends were to him: "Then they sat on the ground with him for seven days and seven nights. No one said a word to him, because they saw how great his suffering was" (Job 2:13, NIV).

Gifts of Gold

"My past carefully molded and shaped me to grow in a way you saw fit. My experiences were ones you saw useful to mold me - even now. You have showered me with mercy and compassion....we are undeserving, Lord, but we come humbly, asking that you grant us our child..." --Journal Entry

Jason's been a rock for me and often speaks truth into our discussions. God is a God of mercy and forgiveness, not giving us what we deserve, but lavishly blessing us beyond what we could ever imagine! At the beginning of this journey, Jason gave me a nugget of truth I treasure: "God does not expect you to grasp it all today or attain some spiritual position to earn His favor. You already have His favor as His child. He expects us to wake up each day and say, 'I can face whatever comes my way today by God's grace and power.' We take one day at a time!"

That's how I'm living now in this trial and will continue to live. I cannot look ahead in my life and try to imagine it without children or try to figure out how it all works out, because it is then that fear creeps in and grief becomes the driving force. I can turn to Him each moment and believe in His goodness. "Which of you, if your son asks for bread, will give him a stone? Or if he asks for a fish, will give him a snake? If you, then, though you are evil, know how to give good gifts to your children, how much more will your Father in heaven give good gifts to those who ask him?" (Matthew 7:9-11, NIV).

Sadly, that last round of IUI in June 2010 was unsuccessful. We continue on this journey. Some days we wonder if we will ever see our dream fulfilled. This road is wearying, the doctor appointments tiresome, the months of wavering emotions seemingly endless. A reason to be ungrateful or to grumble can always be found. Yet, through it all, God is full of grace and mercy. When I don't think I can face another month of disappointment, God instead gives me the gift of peace and joy. Grace for the moment. Even in the darkness of the trial we can feel the light of God's goodness surrounding us as He reassures us that we will make it through and come out as gold (Job 23:10).

My heart has not changed over the past four years of waiting and longing. I'm still hoping to experience pregnancy and children with the same intensity I had in the beginning. I know our joy at that time will be all the sweeter because of the road we've walked. I continue to ask God to answer us in this way and seek to surrender to His undying love for me, trusting He does have a better plan than I could ever hope for or imagine.

When I think about praying and wonder at times if I should continue asking God for the same request, I think of the persistent widow going before the judge in Luke 18. Purely because she persevered in her requests, they were granted. Her faith and persistence changed her heart and her situation. I know many of us do not feel we can ask any harder than we already are, but I will continue to ask God to hear and answer me for this long-awaited child. I hope and pray you have the faith to keep asking too.

"God knew what He was doing from the very beginning. He decided from the outset to shape the lives of those who love Him along the same lines as the life of his Son... After God made that decision of what His children should be like, He followed it up by calling people by name. After He called them by name, He set them on a solid basis with Himself. And then, after getting them established, He stayed with them to the end, GLORIOUSLY COMPLETING what He had begun" Romans 8:29-30 (The Message Bible).

TO THE LIMIT

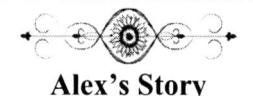

Alex's Story

HERE I sit with a blank page and it's hard to start. How do I translate into words on a page the incredible intensity of feelings the fertility journey brings? I hope you will sense some of those feelings as you read this chapter, and for those of you on this journey, I hope to bring something you can relate to and draw hope from.

I am not a professional writer and have never shared my story in writing, so hopefully you will see past my mistakes and into my heart.

First I would like to share a bit about who I am and what I believe, because such things help define our journeys and will help you understand mine. I grew up in a fairly standard family of mum, dad, and three kids. Mum and Dad loved God, so I grew up knowing God as my Maker and Jesus as my Savior. Through all my experiences I have never doubted the sovereignty of God, only His view of me. I have occasionally doubted such a great God would take the time to consider and love my small life among the billions who exist. I guess I have wondered if I am precious to Him.

Yet in my struggles in life and in my doubting times, God has slowly grown my faith in Him. One of my favorite authors, Philip Yancey, once said that "without great doubt there is no great faith." In trying to create a family, this statement has truly been tested. Life is a journey, and mine is still a work in progress. This story is only my life in part; God has a lot more for me yet.

I would like to start with the hopes and dreams I had for my life when I married my childhood sweetheart, Brent, at the age of twenty. I imagined we would have a perfect family with two or four children, probably not three! I chose nursing as a career because it seemed as though it would work in well with having a family. Brent and I decided we would have children early, knowing they were a gift and blessing from God.

So when I turned twenty-two, we began trying to get pregnant. We were so excited about our decision. I had absolutely no doubt that this was going to be easy for us. Every month I looked for the signs that I was pregnant. I even saw some and would start to make plans. But every month I wasn't. As the months went by, doubt began to grow. At first I didn't want to voice it to Brent because that would make it real. When I did, the doubt got worse.

After going to our family doctor for a raft of tests that all came back fine, I couldn't understand what was going on. It was starting to affect every part of my life...my work and my relationship with Brent, because everything seemed to revolve around getting pregnant. It affected my relationship with God because He seemed to have abandoned me even when I was serving my heart out for Him.

It was so tiring dealing with several grief cycles--the immediate cycle that every month we hadn't conceived and the prospect that we may not be able to conceive at all. I had so many mixed emotions and was unable to define the feelings I had. It was very difficult to celebrate when family and friends became pregnant. I didn't know if I felt happy for them, jealous, or mad. Only those who have walked this road can understand what you go through. Even your husband walks a different journey.

Every month that went by with another period my anxiety levels rose to new heights. I couldn't bring myself to contemplate that

Brent and I may have an issue. Biologically everything was normal for me, and my siblings seemed to be able to get pregnant at the drop of a hat. Brent and I loved each other, loved God, lived our lives as good people with good motives, and would make great parents. There couldn't possibly be anything fair or even godly about us having difficulties with conception. I didn't talk to anyone about our difficulties conceiving, not even Brent. It was as though we thought that if we ignored it the problem would go away.

Finally after about eighteen months, we decided Brent should go for a test. When our family doctor told us Brent's sperm count results were negative, for a minute I thought that meant there was nothing wrong. In actuality the result meant there was never going to be any chance that we could have children, as Brent had been diagnosed with a variant Cystic Fibrosis gene, which caused him to not have vas deferens. This means that although sperm is generated, the tube which carries it to where it is needed is missing. At the time science could offer us nothing to rectify the issue.

I felt numb. I wasn't angry or sad, I wasn't anything. Basically, if I stayed with Brent, I would never get pregnant, and we would never have children together. Brent and I were devastated. I don't think we were capable of processing this together, seeking help, or at that stage even trusting that God loved us enough to help us. We were just working on surviving together.

It was another three months before Brent and I could share this with our families and pastor. It was like a denial; if we didn't face this it wouldn't be real. It was weird, but during this time the verse, "Before I formed you in the womb I knew you" (Jeremiah 1:5 NIV) kept coming to my mind, and I couldn't understand what God was trying to say to me. It was like He was adding to my pain. I remember saying, "God, I don't think I can do this, why are you hurting me, don't you love me, what have I done?"

You know, people have a lot to say when you have some devastating news, mostly out of caring motives, sometimes out of a need to make themselves feel better, or any number of other reasons. Things like "this will be a test to see if you stay together," "there must be sin in your lives," and "you need more faith." I don't blame people for this, as no one can understand what the pain is like without actually experiencing it, but it does leave you feeling even more alone and confused. We ended up hearing so many words, we didn't know which were good words, what was from God, and what should've been ignored. At first I was so desperate for something from God that I listened to everything. After a while I was so disappointed I listened to nothing.

When people were praying for each other at church one night, someone said he really felt God was saying He would give us a child and soon. You would think I'd have been so happy with this word but by then I was in such a bad way. I had had so many "words" and disappointments that I just went home and sobbed and then was so angry. I didn't have the faith to believe this could be true. The days just continued to go by. I was probably in the middle of the sad part of the grieving process but I just closed down. When I try to remember those days now I can't.

And yet God was so faithful to me even when I couldn't be to Him. About a year later our pastor came to us with the news that there was a sixteen-year-old girl who had become pregnant and was in a desperate place. She didn't want to keep the baby, nor did she want an abortion, believing that life started at conception. She wanted this baby to have a Christian mum and dad who would love this child. Our pastor asked us to pray about whether we were the right parents for this baby. We met with the birth mother and father right away; she must have been about five months pregnant. I respected the courage it must have taken for such a young girl to decide to carry this child.

Brent knew this was right with God. I was still working through it as I was in a bad place, but hope started to grow. We went through the whole legal process with social welfare and then just waited. I couldn't believe this would really happen for us; I thought the young girl would change her mind at the last minute, or social welfare would say we couldn't adopt her. Brent was so supportive of me and largely carried the burden of faith. I have such deep respect for him. His courage to believe and to risk being hurt gave me courage too.

One morning the phone rang at three a.m. to let us know our baby girl had been born and we were now parents. The next day Brent and I traveled to the hospital to meet our sweet daughter. She was so beautiful. God had known all along that this little girl was meant for our family. As he formed her in the womb, He knew what He had planned for her life and ours, and even for the life of the young girl who made that very courageous decision.

When we picked her up from the hospital and I held her in my arms, I remembered the verse God had given me: "Before I formed you in the womb I knew you," and I knew He had been preparing me for this. If Brent and I had not had fertility issues, would we have little Emma as part of our family, as we were meant to before the beginning of time, before we were even born? God had given her to us as our responsibility, and it was an enormous privilege and honor to be entrusted with this little life.

My faith grew amazingly as I realized we are not the masters of our destiny. When we give our lives over to God, He orders our path, and it is only He who knows what our future holds. If we had conceived a baby what would have happened to our Emma? As she grows up it is so obvious to us and everyone around that we were meant to be a family. She is true evidence of God working in each of our lives and knowing and loving us all in the midst of millions. Even when we don't have the faith to believe in Him, He believes in us.

So after this miracle you would think I'd have enough faith to trust God with our family, but I confess this wasn't what happened. When Emma was two and a half the three of us went to the UK to have an overseas experience before she started school. We ended up staying for six years. While having Emma didn't cure all those normal hormonal and female urges to have a baby, I never went for help to work through the grief. I just poured my whole time and effort into her. It was easy to put grief aside when Emma was a beautiful baby girl.

When my friends started having their second children, all those feelings began rising up inside me again. I couldn't believe it. I felt so bad for still wanting more. I thought I was such a bad Christian; hadn't God given me enough already? I tried ignoring how I felt but it always came out when I was least expecting it. When having coffee with my friends I would have to leave or go to the bathroom because I would sob uncontrollably and couldn't understand why.

I so loved Emma, this wasn't about her at all. When Emma started asking for a baby sister or brother I would have to explain that mummy and daddy couldn't give her one. I would plunge into another bout of sadness and withdraw from everyone. Everything I thought I had dealt with came up again; all my doubts about God and His love for me. I couldn't be thankful just for Emma, I desperately wanted more--to be pregnant, to give Emma the baby sister or brother she wanted. My whole body cried out to be pregnant. God made us with the desire to have children. I became obsessed with the idea and researched how we could do it.

A new medical intervention, ICSI (intracytoplasmic sperm injection), had been developed since our original diagnosis, whereby fertility specialists could take my egg, operate on Brent to remove his sperm, fertilize the egg in a laboratory, and then re-implant it in me. I was now heading for thirty and really desperate to give this a try. At the time it cost about NZ$18,000 a cycle. We decided to give it one cycle and if it didn't work, then it wasn't meant to be.

I took fertility drugs for six months, then Brent endured a horrible operation, and I had my eggs removed. A week later the specialist implanted two embryos that had started to grow. It was so exciting for me, such a high. We had come so far and I just knew it was going to work.

I injected myself twice a day to try to convince my body it was pregnant. When out with a friend four weeks later, certain I was pregnant and very happy, I started to bleed. I told her I had to go home. I went straight to bed and just shut down. When Brent came home from work and I told him I'd lost the embryos he couldn't say anything. From the next day Brent and I didn't talk about it and for a year we just kind of existed. I went on with life with Emma, and Brent went on working. We started to drift apart and didn't say much to each other because there wasn't much to say.

I started to spiral into a very dark place. I drank too much, went out with "friends" too often, and didn't pay a lot of attention to God. I started to think very dangerous thoughts about not being with Brent because maybe someone else would be able to give me a baby. I am ashamed to say I was not a very good mother during this time; I was not really in a sane frame of mind.

I think the fertility drugs affected my hormones and emotional balance. The fertility group I had been a part of never made contact with me after I rang to say I had miscarried, so I had no medical support either. I really wanted to self-destruct. I started playing around with the idea of relationships with other men and in my darkest days almost stepped over the edge and could've made some of the biggest mistakes of my life, but always something held me back. Always there was a voice in my head that said, "You are loved."

I went to Brent and told him our marriage was over unless he agreed to let me get pregnant with the sperm donor program. He was so wonderful about it and said he would look into it and consider it. I could see he was uncomfortable, but I was just so obsessed I didn't care. I pressured him so much and pushed him so hard he just stopped talking to me because it was my only subject of conversation.

One night as we were watching a movie on the couch, having not talked to each other all week, Brent started to cry. He turned to me and said, "I love you." It echoed what God had been trying to say to me in my head. I broke down and sobbed. Brent and I held onto each other and cried. I told him I loved him and something released me. I realized I would have wanted to live my whole life with him even if I had known we couldn't have kids before we got married. I released him from having to consider the donor program and we just thanked God for Emma.

During the following year I went for professional counseling, and Brent and I worked through so many things we had allowed into our lives over the grief from not being able to conceive. I felt that while God hadn't planned for Brent and me not to have children, He is still our Savior, and we are still subject in part to the fallen world we live in.

God took that painful and wrong situation and made it right. He had loved me when I didn't love Him, He had believed in me when I didn't believe in me. He had reminded me of my love for Brent when I had forgotten it and gave me a beautiful child who was just so perfect for us. When I started to work through my grief and emotions I started to see how much God had loved me and how very important my life was to Him.

I am now forty. I do still have emotions about not being pregnant and wanting a baby. I still grieve and probably always will, but it's in balance with what I have, and that is so much more. I will always carry a remnant of sadness with me, but it no longer defines me. I am careful whom I share my journey with, as it can be hard to understand the intense feelings infertility brings without having been there. When Catherine asked if I would share my story I said yes because this book is for those of you on this journey and for those of you walking alongside someone on this journey.

My intention in telling my story is not to provide you with a road map, but to let you know that we are all on a journey and yours is as precious to God as mine is. Each person's story is as unique as the individual involved. Believe it, God does love you.

THE LEAST OF THESE

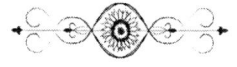

Michelle S's Story

IF only I was younger; hadn't gone to that clairvoyant; was more relaxed; didn't focus on it so much; changed my focus; had more fun. If only people didn't say such well-meaning but essentially unhelpful things: "Perhaps you should have a holiday – some friends of ours got pregnant that way"; "It'll happen when it's meant to happen"; "Have you thought about adopting?"

If only I could've seen ahead. If someone had told me in 2003 that I would get pregnant in 2007 and have a healthy, happy, gorgeous son, perhaps I would have relaxed and made the most of being childless. But then, if we hadn't worked so hard to access fertility treatment, perhaps we would still be trying to get pregnant even now. Seeing ahead might have helped reduce the stress, sadness, depression, envy, panic attacks, and the impact on our sexual relationship.

I can see now that getting pregnant in 2007 and having our baby in 2008 was perfect timing for us as a couple. Life is better now than it was six years ago. But having a crystal ball is not reality, nor is it part of God's plan for our lives. Future-telling can be a dangerous and debilitating tool – it can have the opposite effect and bring death instead, as part of my story highlights.

In a nutshell, it took from November 2003 to November 2007 for my husband and me to conceive a child. Four long years, but for some, the fertility journey can be much longer. When we held our son for the first time we sobbed with a whirlpool of emotion – we were holding our child. He was so worth the wait.

I was 28 in 2000 and married for two years when I thought I should tell my female doctor about a particularly painful period. I was told it was probably a fertile egg and the pain a part of my normal fertility. I had never heard of such a thing, but since I was about two years away from starting a family I just frowned, paid for the odd advice, and walked out of her office. If only...

If only I had fought to have more tests.

Five years later, after trying unsuccessfully to get pregnant for two years, a fertility specialist told me I had suspected endometriosis and would need to go on a waiting list for publicly funded surgery. *Tick-tock, tick-tock.*

Rewind to 1995. A so-called clairvoyant tells me I will marry somebody from the northern hemisphere who hails from the east (check), I will have difficulty getting pregnant (check), and I will have a difficult pregnancy (oh so wrong!). Two years later I hand over my life to God and ask forgiveness for visits to clairvoyants and other activities in the twenty-five years of doing things my way. Two more years later I meet and marry my northern hemisphere Christian man whose father is from India. We move back to New Zealand to start a family and enjoy a blissful married life.

My husband and I were hoping we would get pregnant fairly quickly but after six months and still just the two of us, I was hit by the memory of 1995. Like a tape recorder implanted in my brain, over and over I could hear this voice saying, "You will have difficulty getting pregnant." I held it inside until, nearly bursting from sadness, fear, and guilt, I asked others to help me pray against this "curse." At the same time, I started investigating mild fertility treatment (natural progesterone) and natural family planning (ovulation charting). We were officially on the fertility roller coaster.

At the end of the first year of trying (2004) we moved cities and made an appointment with a fertility specialist shortly after settling in. The thought of having a diagnosis for why we were not getting pregnant made me feel lighter and slightly hopeful. It would cancel out the guesswork but might bring its own stresses of finding out how to remedy the issue. I was also nervous that the problem might not be with me but with my husband. That fear was quickly put to rest when the specialist said, "He should be proud of himself. You should tell him to frame these results!" If I had allowed such things he very well would have!

After a couple of examinations I was told I had probable endometriosis and was put on the waiting list for laparoscopic surgery. Ten months later grade-two endometriosis was removed and we were left to try again. Apparently you are meant to be quite fertile after such surgery. I guess it happens for some and not others, as no pregnancy ensued.

During 2005 and 2006 we worked hard, saving for a deposit on a house, cementing friendships, and settling into our new community, all the while trying to get pregnant naturally, supernaturally, and medically. We put up our hands for a Lipiodol Flush trial (flushing out my fallopian tubes with poppy seed oil), which has apparently produced positive results for those with unexplained infertility and endometriosis. Again my chances of getting pregnant in the next three months were really high. My tubes were clear and my endometriosis was only grade two, so the fertility clinic said our infertility must be unexplained rather than due to a specific issue. They also said thirty-three was young so not to panic about my age.

After two unsuccessful IUIs, we took another step down the natural-fertility path recommended by a friend from church. My fertility naturopath picked up on candida, a low positive lupus result (my immune system could be attacking our fertilized eggs), a leaky gut, causing mal-absorption of essential minerals and vitamins, and intolerance to wheat and dairy. All could contribute to endometriosis and why we were not getting pregnant. Believing that a healthy body can help create a healthy baby, I began treating my symptoms with a change in diet, increased exercise, and specific herbs. I certainly felt better physically.

By this time the list of friends who were pregnant reached double figures. It was getting harder and harder to hide our pain. Each infertile month was like a kick in the stomach, and when friends with one or two children started announcing second and third pregnancies we almost packed up and went overseas! People's prayers, hugs, and empathetic ears weren't diminishing our empty-nest emotions. We also began to feel insecure at the place where we thought we should feel safest – church.

Church is a great breeding place, and the focus on family meant we felt like outsiders. After one–too-many pregnant bellies and a near panic attack, we decided to take a break from services. It's been five years since we've been part of a church family, but we are still connected on an almost daily basis with Christian friends.

Staying away from church services was not entirely connected to our infertility journey. We were burnt out before we started trying to get pregnant. Our weekends were increasingly taken up by house hunting and working, and we were physically exhausted. Most importantly, as we spent almost every spare evening and weekend doing church-related things with the same people, we were living in an insular Christian bubble rather than relating to the wider community or spending time with other friends and family.

Church was becoming bigger than our relationship with God. Rather than formally meeting on a Sunday, we met in small groups. We knew we needed to take time out at such an important stage of our lives.

I don't think I lived in the "why me, why us?" place for long, if at all, as I had a deep sense we would eventually get pregnant. The issue was always when. My diary records moments of "I guess it's God's timing" but in all honesty, I didn't believe it. I believed we were ready. We had done the "right" things and honored God by putting Him and our marriage first.

We worked hard to cement a strong relationship built on friendship, faith, honesty, and personal development so we would not repeat the mistakes of our parents. We both come from broken, dysfunctional families and were determined to change history and have a marriage worth celebrating in years to come.

When the desires of my heart seemed to be falling on deaf ears, I ended up pushing God away. I shut Him out and was determined not to let the words of 1995 ring true. In hindsight I wanted to prove to God that I could make it happen – if He was going to take His time, then I would show Him we could get pregnant without Him, in our time. I thought I was ready for the battle; looking back, I only got the stuffing knocked out of me.

In the third quarter of 2006 my body went into stress overload mode. I came out in itchy bumps all over my body. We were house sitting in a cold, damp house while the home we loved was in the conditional offer process. I was juggling three jobs. Being on the IVF waiting list gave us hope.

In January 2007 we moved into our first house, and after eight years of marriage I could nest and make a home for our incomplete family. My doctor called to say we would probably start IVF in April, so the year ahead looked promising.

In the lead up to IVF I wasn't spending much time with God. I could sense Him behind me but we didn't talk much, or rather I chose not to listen. I relaxed the special diet and took a break from the herbs as money was a little tight, but I was feeling healthy and a bit more positive about my fertility.

At times the pressure of trying to get pregnant got to both of us and manifested itself in deep sadness, anger, envy, panic, and desperation. We took the odd month off trying and worked on bringing some romance and intimacy into the bedroom! Hard to do when utterly exhausted. Mostly we flopped into bed and snuggled for comfort and warmth.

D-Day for starting IVF was approaching. It was time to change the focus from trying to get pregnant naturally to letting science help us. We were excited about the possibility of getting pregnant but nervous about the IVF process and the chance it might not work. After acupuncture, popping various vitamins and minerals, herbal tonics, prayer, and lost sleep, we hopped on board the IVF train.

I was torn between letting go and still trying. I thought that if I stopped trying God would say, "No, it's not going to happen – ever," or my momentum would wane and I would crash and burn. I wanted to keep going to remain in control of the situation.

I wrote in my diary, "What if I embark on this journey with God and He doesn't answer our prayers during IVF? How will I feel? What will I believe about God? How can I believe in something that doesn't work? What will that say/mean/look like to friends and family who don't believe in God?"

If I didn't let go I wondered if God would deprive me of my desire to be a mum. If I did let go and stopped panicking, perhaps I would be free to accept my barrenness, something I didn't want to do.

Despite the inner spiritual struggles we had a great IVF experience. The drug taking and needle injecting went smoothly, with no adverse side effects. I produced nine eggs and all nine fertilized. Five made it to day three, of those five, only three made it to day five (blastocysts). We were proud parents of three microscopic beings. We thanked God for his blessings and small miracles. We believed God ordained life.

The first transfer was in June. Apparently, the embryo was one of the best they had seen! They froze the other two embryos. With a skip in our step we went home to wait the dreaded two weeks to see if I was pregnant.

It was a confusing fortnight. In the early days I felt twinges of what could be the embryo implanting. But as the days wore on I felt the familiar hollow and barren sensations of my approaching period. I prepared myself for a negative result by talking and crying lots. The nurse who called with bad news must have thought I was very brave and stoical for not crying. If only she could have seen me seconds after I hung up.

We were devastated. I was disappointed in my body for rejecting or failing to accept the almost perfect embryo. What more did God want? What did I have to do to get Him to bless my body and gift us with a child? I was desperate.

Like Job, Esther, and Elijah (in the bible), I had questions; most of them went unanswered. The negative result broke our hearts but understanding that sorrow is normal, we tenderly and patiently picked each other up and continued walking the infertile path.

On the recommendation of our IVF support group, we had booked a week on a topical island after the first transfer. The holiday and timing were perfect. Aside from the fact that we relaxed, slept, and ate our way out of sadness, we also had fun together. Something we hadn't done for a while.

On returning home I focused on my health, doing all I could to prepare my body for another embryo transfer. My naturopath wanted me to wait about six months. I compromised and waited two. My patience was wearing thin.

Weeks before the next transfer (August, 2007), I asked a close friend if she could gather some people together for a prayer session. One other woman was about to embark on a round of IVF. The prayer time was amazing and as a group we continue to meet and pray for women going through infertility issues.

The next transfer was devastatingly negative. We were tired, discouraged, and asking ourselves "Where to from here?" We had one embryo left. If that didn't work we would need to go through another round of IVF, which we were told would be in August 2008. I would be thirty-six and still young, but not young enough for our liking.

I knew I couldn't block God out anymore. My strength was running low and the sadness was affecting me on many levels. I wrote in my diary that I wanted to approach the next few months differently. I wanted to walk with God. After reading Zechariah 4:6 I wrote: "Not by the resources of many or one. It will not be by my cleverness, my ability, or my physical strength that I will get pregnant, have a baby, or be happy, but by the Spirit of God."

I asked myself what that scripture actually means: "Not by might nor by power, but by my Spirit, says the Lord." Is keeping fit and healthy, using the last frozen blastocyst and going for the next round of free IVF doing it by my might and power? Perhaps "by my Spirit" means letting go and not doing anything, just letting it happen naturally – allowing God to give life in His timing. Ouch.

In reflection I wrote how I had continually come unstuck through my independence, need for control, and "I can do it" attitude. The theme of my life was quite apparent, and God spoke clearly about letting Him take control. This was easier said than done. But with God, and occasional help from my husband and a pastor friend, I worked on issues over the next few months and felt something shift inside.

One of the pivotal things I worked on was changing my motivation for getting myself healthy – physically and spiritually. I realized I needed to get healthy for me, full stop; not to have a child, although that would be a great result. I wanted to do it so I could live my life to the potential God had created in me.

The other life-changing issue was facing my fears and asking God to help me overcome them. I feared I was going to die. I wrote in my diary "perhaps this fear is debilitating and subconsciously stopping me from wanting to get pregnant?" Deep down I thought I would die in childbirth or pregnancy. Writing it down was a revelation, and over the course of the year I worked on overcoming this fear.

Others began to notice a change in my countenance: an inner peace. The spiritual work was long lasting and had deep consequences.

The burden of being infertile and not having a child in our life was so big at times. We had to consider the fact that we might not have children of our own flesh and blood, but it never sat well with us. We were definitely keen to adopt or foster if after a point we hadn't conceived, but we knew we hadn't reached that point. As more and more babies were being born around us, we felt isolated and different. We coped by becoming protective of our relationship and personal free time, perhaps to the detriment of friendships, but we felt that true friends would understand and be there for us at the other end.

Two days before the third and final transfer in late November 2007, I felt nervous, apprehensive, and numb. I didn't want to get my hopes up, but I also wanted to be optimistic. I felt the timing was perfect, but I wasn't sure God felt the same way.

I wrote a prayer, "God I ask that you hear me, that you bless my body, that you heal me from ill health, from infertility. God help me to grow during this time, to wise up, to mature, to strengthen in personality and character. God help me heal and get through this season."

Transfer day came a day after my father's birthday and thirty-four years to the day after I was conceived. It was exciting that the embryo survived the thawing, but it was weakest of the three. The first was beautiful, according to the fertility clinic, and the second won an award for being the best looking embryo of the week, which was hard to deal with as they didn't result in a baby. This transfer was like the first two; we were told it had been textbook and were lovingly sent home to wait.

Again I experienced the confusing PMT/early pregnancy signals. Tender breasts from day one and period pain twinges but a week early. I went from being mildly excited at the start to completely deflated five days later. On Sunday I bought myself a sexy lingerie set and wore it proudly but sadly. My slightly PMT-sized breasts looked great!

A couple of days before the blood test I started spotting and was convinced it hadn't worked. So much stronger this time around, I started dreaming about fun things we could do between November 2007 and August 2008 when we would most likely be starting round two of IVF.

I rang to tell the clinic I was spotting, which meant my period was coming and I would take the test a day early. In the afternoon I saw the clinic had called but chose to ignore the message. At the end of the day I went home, made myself a cup of tea, and sat on the couch, ready to watch an episode of my favorite soap while I listened to the message alone.

Moments later I was hysterical and by myself at that! The nurse was telling me I was pregnant! When I rang my husband at work I don't think he could understand me at first. I was laughing and crying so much he started doing the same. Obviously a happy phone call, it could only mean one thing.

There was much to celebrate that night. This was our first positive pregnancy test in four years! We wanted to hold it lightly for fear of it ending in miscarriage. When I started spotting almost a month later on Christmas Eve I was told to go to bed immediately and rest for at least an hour. It was a tearful start to the holidays and a very horizontal Christmas Day. I have never had so much attention. My grandparents and parents didn't let me lift a finger. I was carrying precious cargo and they sure let me know it.

To cut a long story short, our weakest embryo turned out to be the strongest of the three and we had an amazing pregnancy together. My body responded well to carrying our child and I loved every moment of it. The first twenty weeks were wracked with the fear of miscarriage, but we celebrated every milestone (eight, twelve, and twenty week scans) and broadcast our results to all we knew.

So many dear friends had lost babies in the first trimester and I was afraid our little miracle could be taken away from us. Apparently it's quite common for pregnant women to fear death, be it their own, the baby's, or their husband's. Thanks to raging hormones, sometimes these fears were quite consuming, but with the help of husband, family, friends, God, and books, I was able to push them aside and relish my beautiful pregnancy.

I knew from conception that we had a son. Theodore (Gift from God) Reuben (see, a Son) Adam (earth, man) was born August 14, 2008 after an amazing labor (not too long, not too quick). I was able to claim my body back from medical interventions for fertility treatment with a drug-free water birth. Thanks to some serious research and reading *Supernatural Childbirth* by Jackie Mize, the pain was manageable, and my midwives said I was the calmest, most relaxed woman they had seen giving birth in years.

My husband and I were so proud of ourselves, and more so of our amazingly beautiful son. He was a true gift from God and we have been in awe of him ever since. At the time of writing this, he is fourteen months old and a beautiful child inside and out.

We still don't understand why we had to wait so long to get pregnant. Unexplained infertility is an unhelpful label to carry and we still ache in memory of those four roller coaster years. It has scarred us in different ways. My husband is still confused by the "why."

I have lost some of the sting, being caught up in the now and future with our son, but my heart breaks when I hear of other difficult journeys to gain a child. I also wonder how I will react when we try for child number two. We have chosen to try naturally for our second child and at this stage will not pay for a second round of IVF. We want to trust and believe in God.

We both love God and do our best to walk with Him. We are truly grateful for the gift of our son and the blessed lives we live. We also understand that the infertility journey is a process. In all honesty, having Theo has not completed our healing, but we are slowly getting there. We are moving into a time of restoration.

The last entry in my diary on the day I found out I was pregnant is, "Do not be anxious about anything, but in every situation, by prayer and petition, with thanksgiving, present your requests to God. And the peace of God, which transcends all understanding, will guard your hearts and your minds in Christ Jesus" (Philippians 4:6-7, NIV). I read this scripture daily throughout my pregnancy.

MODERN DAY MIRACLES

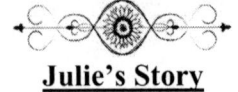

Julie's Story

IAN and I married in 1992. Already in our thirties, it wasn't long before we decided to start a family. We thought it would happen automatically, within a couple months or so. Little did we realize how wrong we would be. Months and months went by and much to our dismay, no pregnancy was forthcoming.

After a year, I visited my gynecologist and underwent many tests to try and find out why things weren't progressing. No major problem was found, apart from a small amount of endometriosis. After surgery for this, my gynecologist said my chances of becoming pregnant would improve. Ian and I took off overseas for a couple of months, having been told it would probably just happen, maybe while we were away enjoying ourselves!

We continued to try, and still nothing. As the months turned into years the more upsetting it became. Each month was a time of grieving this very private grief. It is strange grieving for something that has not even existed. No one around me seemed to have any idea how it felt.

Even a visit to the local shopping mall was upsetting; seeing young mothers, often teenagers, pushing around their babies. Sometimes I would leave in floods of tears. Every time a friend became pregnant, it felt like a knife going through my heart. I was pleased for them but ached inside, particularly when one of my closest friends married and had her first baby ten months later.

Meeting new people became an uneasy experience, as often their first question would be, "Have you any children?" I never liked this, especially when they asked whether it was my choice or whether I couldn't get pregnant! It was such a personal matter.

In due time we had more medical investigations. Nothing unusual turned up. We just prayed and prayed. We sought prayer and counsel from our pastor and searched our hearts for any spiritual blockage. We wondered if perhaps it was not on God's agenda for us to have children. Maybe we needed to surrender this to Him? Perhaps His purpose for us as a couple didn't include children? If that were the case, we just wanted to get on with it. We didn't want to waste our sorrows.

But as we prayed we had a deep conviction that we were meant to be parents. God spoke to us through a number of scriptures in our daily readings so we continued to pray, believing it to be according to His will.

We decided to become involved with respite foster care through a Christian agency. Not only would it give us experience, we could make the most of our waiting time by channeling our love to needy children in the community. It was challenging yet deeply rewarding. We were always given the option of taking on each case, but even so we found ourselves thrown in the deep end, sometimes with children from very desperate backgrounds. Many of them just loved being in a home doing normal family things like "helping Dad" in the garage and washing the car – things we take for granted can be novelties for some. Our biggest challenge was an abused ten-year-old who was emotionally disturbed.

More than four years went by. There were good days and bad days. Often when one of us was struggling, the other would be strong and vice versa. We kept on encouraging one another. I remember one particularly difficult Saturday when I was crying out to God about the situation. Why, when we felt we were meant to be parents, was nothing happening? I opened my Bible and the following verse from Jeremiah spoke clearly to me: "I am the LORD, the God of all mankind. Is anything too hard for me?" (Jeremiah 32:27, NIV)

The following Sunday the prayer healing team stood at the front of our church and read out some inspired words for individuals in the congregation. One was for a "barren woman." "God wants you to know that nothing is too hard for Him" – the very scripture God had given me the day before. I was stunned. It was such an encouragement to keep hanging in there.

Time went on. Through yet another medical investigation, we finally discovered something obscure relating to my husband which was believed to be causing the problem. A morphology test measuring the ratio of the length to the width of the sperm revealed that although the sperm count and motility were good, the morphology was not. The sperm were almost all the wrong shape, which caused an inability to penetrate the egg. The experts told us it was irreversible, which was quite a bombshell. Our only hope (and a slim one at that) was IVF using the ICSI (intracytoplasmic sperm injection) method. At this point we went to the eldership and requested specific prayer for the problem.

Our pastor and elders came to pray with us, specifically addressing that cause. It was a great encouragement. We determined we would wait a couple of months and if nothing happened, then try IVF.

A few weeks later, God spoke again to me from Ezekiel 12:27-28 (NIV): "Son of man, the house of Israel is saying, 'The vision he sees is for many years from now, and he prophesies about the distant future.' Therefore say to them, 'This is what the Sovereign Lord says: None of my words will be delayed any longer, whatever I say will be fulfilled, declares the Sovereign Lord.'"

It was just as the scripture said. That very month, within three months of the pastor and elders' prayers, and without having to undergo IVF, I was pregnant What a miracle – nothing is impossible with God. We were absolutely ecstatic.

The pregnancy went well and we were so blessed by the arrival of our beautiful daughter who weighed in at 6lb 3oz. She's a true miracle and we are privileged to be her parents.

When she was just eight months old, I discovered I was pregnant again - amazing considering our medical situation.

Unfortunately that pregnancy ended early in miscarriage. A few months later I had another early miscarriage. We had more prayer and conceived for a third time. Everything seemed to be going well in the first few weeks, but when we went to have a scan there was no heartbeat. We were absolutely devastated. I went to hospital for a D and C. Even though the baby definitely had not survived, I felt they were taking my baby away from me. It took quite a while to get over the grief.

Despite having lost these three babies, it was amazing that I had actually conceived after being told there was no chance. After another morphology test my husband was told that the original problem, supposedly irreversible, had disappeared and he was normal! God had done a miraculous healing work, but we still kept losing the babies. I was now over forty, and the medical fact is that one in every two pregnancies miscarry when the mother is this age.

Following the D and C we continued trying for another child but nothing happened. We went back to the fertility clinic and had three attempts at a treatment, AIH (artificial insemination by husband). Although my body produced a good number of eggs, all attempts failed.

We still believed we were supposed to have another child. Ian had a real struggle at this point. After all we had been through, he found it difficult to believe that God would taunt us with such clear promises and not fulfill them. He couldn't understand why God seemed to be delaying His promise. He felt strongly that if God was to deliver His promise, then He wanted us to pray specifically about the child and give the child a name. And so Ian did.

Time passed and I became so tired of praying. For me time wasn't running out, it had already run out, and I had to move on with my life. I set a date and told the Lord I wasn't going to pray about it after that. That date came and I surrendered it. I had to trust God. Even though the complete promise seemed unfulfilled, I had to trust in His sovereignty. I was so thankful and grateful for the lovely little girl God had given us and accepted that if we had only one child, then that was absolutely fine.

Bringing some finality and closure was difficult, but it was helpful for me and I did move on. Our daughter started school and I went back to work part time. I became involved in worship leading at church and taught Bible in schools. Life was good and we were so grateful to God for what we had. But even though I'd stopped praying, now our little daughter was asking God for a brother or sister!

In April 2003 a couple of remarkable things happened. After church one Sunday morning a friend said she'd had a vivid dream in which I told her I was pregnant. I just laughed! I was quickly reminded of someone in the Bible who laughed after being told she would have a baby in her old age – Sarah (Genesis 18:12).

I thought about my friend's dream a lot that week. My period was due but it hadn't arrived. We had stocktaking at work that Saturday. I kept thinking "what if?" and must admit I was a little careful not to overdo things, just in case. Also during that week, the scripture God had given me for our daughter, "none of my words will be delayed any longer," popped back into my readings. The following Monday I was still overdue. Just to put my mind to rest I bought a pregnancy test and was blown away when it was positive. I was forty-six years old.

The day I found out I was pregnant, I overheard our daughter talking to a school friend in the bedroom. Her friend asked, "Is your mummy going to give you a baby?" Our daughter replied indignantly, "No! God's going to give us a baby!" She had absolutely no idea about our news. The experience was quite amazing – it was like a prophecy from a child. We didn't tell her until I was fifteen weeks pregnant.

After finding out, I immediately contacted the local Recurrent Miscarriage Clinic, having previously been under their care. I was told not to get my hopes up. With my situation and age, statistically it was almost impossible to conceive and there was only a 2 to 4% chance that the baby would ever develop a heartbeat.

But the following week at our scan, there was the baby's heart, beating strongly. We were overjoyed. However we were told we had a high chance of losing the baby and continued to be scanned each week.

At about nine weeks the clinic told me we had reached a high risk point for miscarrying. I went to the Lord again, as I was feeling very anxious. In my readings for that day from the book Jeremiah, a couple of scriptures spoke directly to me: "For He did not kill me in the womb" (Jeremiah 20:17, NIV).

I felt I'd lost so many years waiting for a family, so I asked God about it. He gave me Joel 2:25 (NIV): "I will repay you for the years the locusts have eaten."

The pregnancy continued. Apart from terrible morning sickness, apparently a good sign, there were no problems. At about the thirteen-week mark I started to relax as the major danger period was over. At thirty-five weeks, the obstetrician at the high-risk clinic said to me, "In cases like yours, we expect the worst and hope for the best. It looks like we are going to get the best." I felt a sense of contentment and peace. In the last few weeks I anxiously monitored movement and had a couple of visits to the hospital to check when things were quiet. With older mothers the placenta sometimes fails towards the end of pregnancy.

I was induced at thirty-nine weeks because of this risk, and on December 2, 2003, our son was born weighing 9lb 1oz. His name, Matthew, means "Gift of God," and that is what he is. It is the name of Ian's dearly beloved Granddad and the name Ian gave this child when he was challenged to pray some years earlier.

The nurse in charge told me that in all the years she had been running the Recurrent Miscarriage Clinic (sixteen years or so), I was the oldest mum under their care who had had a successful natural pregnancy without the use of donor eggs.

Our daughter, now twelve, loves music and dance; our son is a bubbly five-year-old schoolboy.

We are so grateful to God for what He has done, not only for giving us the miracle of having our family, but also for the deep work He has done in our hearts and lives through this process. He has changed us inside. Even though the hard places aren't pleasant, we're thankful for the lessons we've been able to learn there.

We're really grateful He has kept our marriage strong. It was not always easy; maintaining good communication was a key.

We're also grateful for the people who supported us by praying. It has been so vital and encouraging, and we're humbled by their faithfulness.

Just after our son was born, our daughter said, "I KNEW we'd have a baby, Mum." I asked her, "Why is that?" She replied, "Because we prayed and prayed and prayed."

THE CURSE IS BROKEN

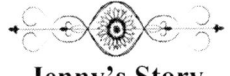

Jenny's Story

OUT the other side of my long valley of miscarriages I am more aware of how our lives are so much about seasons. Now I can only try to recapture the sense of what it was like in retrospect, and it feels very different than my blessed life with two daughters.

I was working as a midwife in Brighton, England, when I started trying to have children. I was devastated when I started bleeding at thirteen weeks in my first pregnancy, and a scan showed my baby had died at nine weeks. My grief was immense and doubly brutal, as at work I had to give evidence on a baby's death from an extremely rare complication following a doctor's ventouse delivery. Angry parents and my own burdens felt unbearably heavy. We named our baby Meredith and sent her on her spiritual journey as we floated a handpicked posy of wild flowers down Barcombe River in Sussex.

Two further miscarriages later (the pain slightly less each time but the resignation twice as strong) I was referred to the Recurrent Miscarriage Clinic at St Mary's Hospital in London. I came away with wet pants from bursting my bladder trying to get off the scan bed after refusing to let a rather determined doctor take a high vaginal swab. This is a usual procedure when investigating miscarriages, but I didn't want it done then.

They also didn't approve of my not wanting to be included in their then experimental work (now well established) with heparin, an anti-coagulant drug sometimes used in pregnancy. Instead I went on low-dose aspirin and fish oil tablets to treat my new diagnosis of anti-phospholipid syndrome. With this condition, the unusually sticky platelets cause blood clots in the tiny spiral arteries of the uterus, blocking oxygen and nutrients from getting to the developing fetus.

The treatment worked, as I became pregnant with my now twelve-year-old daughter, but I will always believe the real cause of my blessing was God's work. Years later my obstetrician questioned whether anti-phospholipid syndrome was the main cause of my miscarriages or just an underlying fluctuating condition.

Prior to this pregnancy I would go walking, tuning into my profound sense of doom and despair about not having any control over that part of my life. I, of all people! I had to be one of the healthiest people on the planet – vegetarian for many years, fit, informed. Growing into an adult in the '80s had given me a feministic sense of control and power over my life. I was a planner, careful and precise, and this wasn't supposed to happen. I was helpless.

My father had died some years earlier when I was twenty-four, so I couldn't borrow strength from him anymore when things like this happened. I started to tune into the need for a heavenly Father. One who was bigger than I, bigger than my human frailty. Out walking through one valley of darkness, I wandered into a high Anglican church. Inside, it was richly inlaid with gilt mosaic walls and iconic art. I stood beside one of the many statue saints, lit a candle, and paid my money for it. Although I grew up a Presbyterian, I thought "This will do," and asked God to meet me where I left off back when I was sixteen or seventeen. I started praying the Lord's Prayer every day, mainly as I couldn't think of how to talk to God otherwise. I focused intently on each line and was amazed at how all-encompassing and connecting it was. I now had a lifeline to cling to.

My pregnancy continued wonderfully, culminating in the powerful and beautiful home birth of my oldest daughter. Tragically, when she was nearly three, my marriage broke up. When my daughter was one and a half, we moved to New Zealand at about the same time that I became a born-again Christian. There foll-owed moving house two times, and returning to work, as well as becoming firmly rooted in a wonderful church. Three years later I remarried and we started hoping for another child. I thought, "No problem. I'll just take my aspirin and fish oil tablets and it will be fine." But it wasn't. I went on to have ten more miscarriages over the course of three years.

Having had an emotionally challenging childhood, I was quite good at enduring disappointment and so coped reasonably well even though it was extremely difficult. Despite a probable shock response of feeling cold and numb, I was encouraged by Romans 5:3-4 (NIV): "...suffering produces perseverance; perseverance, character; and character, hope." I believed there would be a baby at the end as a reward for all the learning. The Recurrent Miscarriage Clinic program, this time in Auckland, New Zealand, was intended to give hope and encouragement, but I grew to fear the scans that always crushed my dreams and my spirit.

Many people were praying for me: my church home group, people in church whom I sat beside, altar calls, the Pastoral Care team. The Pastoral Prayer team was incredible. They fasted in prayer for me, sent flowers, lent me CDs and books--*Jesse Found In Heaven* by Pastor Chris Pringle being one of them. It revealed to me the continued life of our children in heaven. On one altar call a pastor directed me to look up the scriptures, "'Sing, barren woman, you who never bore a child; burst into song, shout for joy, you who were never in labor; because more are the children of the desolate woman than of her who has a husband,' says the Lord. 'Enlarge the place of your tent, stretch your tent curtains wide, do not hold back; lengthen your cords, strengthen your stakes. For you will spread out to the right and to the left; your descendants will dispossess nations and settle in their desolate cities'" (Isaiah 54:1-3, NIV).

I read it over and over again, trying to understand. Eventually it spoke reams to me and I clung to its truth, because all scripture is truth. To me, the barren woman was the miscarrying woman whose husband deserted her (as still happens in some cultures, even our own). Her children were "more" because they were being parented in heaven and they were "more" because more were on their way into the world. What a privilege to have had those babies who were now holy heirs in heaven. We indeed enlarged the place of our tent by adding another bedroom and bathroom to our house well before the miracle pregnancy came along. It was an opportunity to do what we could in an earthly way to help our mission.

Capable of faith and spiritually strong, I was physically weak from forever going through the first trimester of pregnancies, anemic from blood loss. Usually I needed an operation to remove the dead fetus, having hung on to the pregnancies for a further six weeks. All those general anesthetics! Once I went into respiratory arrest and needed resuscitating when my oxygen saturations took a nosedive. Interestingly I'd had a ghastly, dark, foreboding as I went under anesthesia.

I felt exposed, literally, by being half-naked on the operating table in front of people I worked with. Staff can often be in that situation, and we try to be pragmatic, but it's not always easy. What with my spiritual exploration and growth through this time I had become quite experienced at being "stripped down" before God as well as those interceding for me in prayer, but it is never a comfortable experience. I felt stripped down and exposed in every facet of my being – physical, emotional, mental, and spiritual.

Another learning curve was dealing with a niggling fear at the back of my head that God might be punishing me for my previous sins. I had to make myself grasp hold of the fact that God does not cause suffering to justify sin. Christ has paid the price for us. God teaches and guides His sons and daughters because He wants us to be blessed. It is not His character to be punitive when we fail. He only loves us and wants us to succeed. I knew all this but had to keep adjusting myself mentally whenever that cruel thought crept into my mind.

For some miscarriages I chose to remain away from the hospital, and they were bloody and painful ordeals. Once when we were camping, I had to make many trips across the green to the toilets, eventually staying there for three hours! Cold, in early shock, covered in blood and in excruciating pain, fortunately I was alone. My husband and daughter had gone fishing. By the time they came back I was composed. When this happened for the ninth time and while we were staying at my mum's during our house renovations, I decided enough was enough, I wouldn't try again. But the next morning, just as I stepped through the door of the shower, I sensed very strongly that it would be okay to. I realized this was a heart desire. It was my mind that had been calculating not to, but my heart said "try." I remember my senior pastor saying desires of the heart are God-inspired and therefore dreams that will come true because they are in keeping with His will. Excited by this memory, I believed I was onto a winner. I just didn't know when.

After another miscarriage I decided to have an IUCD (contraceptive device) fitted at the same time as my operation to give me a rest from pregnancy – I was worried about becoming too anemic. I became pregnant so easily. I couldn't use the contraceptive pill, as I had a greater tendency to clot because of my slight anti-phospholipid syndrome. In hospital awaiting my operation, not a single person entered the room for four hours. I turned to God in prayer, and after four awesome hours in the Spirit I knew everything was going to be all right.

Around this time someone in the church visiting from Africa prayed for me against the spirit of miscarriage. I wondered what he meant and thought it was a bit witch doctorish. Another person known to have a gift of prophecy hinted at a curse of rejection and even self-rejection. Thinking back to the times in childhood when my sister had practiced voodoo on my baby doll, I thought it was possible, albeit wacky.

At that time my husband Andrew and I embarked on a Cleansing Stream course. The ramifications for my life were miraculous, far–reaching, and everlasting. This six-month course, authored by learned theologians and pastors from America, involves study, prayer, watching a monthly DVD, and attending a weekend retreat at the end. It deals with spiritually bound areas of one's life that are resulting in physical, emotional, spiritual, and mental ill health. We had been too busy with other church activities to do it before then, but as it transpired, this was God's perfect timing. It was the first time the course had addressed the issue of freemasonry.

Freemasonry is an old order originating in Europe. The members were builders and stonemasons for the temples and cathedrals of Europe during the Middle Ages. Later the organization took on more of a relaxation and social function. It is an exclusive brotherhood, exercising total secrecy. Many heads of state in America are freemasons, for instance. On the outside, it appears an upright club that does voluntary acts to help the community.

According to previous masters of the lodge who broke away and became Christians, those who climb the leadership ladder swear up to thirty-three oaths of allegiance at bizarre occult ceremonies for each of the thirty-three positions of leadership they reach. It is hard to understand how people would make oaths, which ostensibly are curses on one's own family's health. I can only surmise that they don't believe there is really any power in what they are saying, thinking it is just a quaint, traditional ceremony and go along with it in good humor. My grandfather and great-grandfather were masters of their lodge, the level at which curses on women's reproductive organs are made. Andrew thinks his Scottish grandparents were also involved with freemasonry.

Andrew and I really applied ourselves to this course. We felt it was the last thing we hadn't yet done to try and help ourselves grow spiritually and have God's blessing on our lives. Finally being able to release my mess "as is" to God was a major breakthrough. I started to look different. My broken face no longer looked broken when I caught a glimpse of it in a mirror or shop window.

For the previous six months I had been deeply broken, tender-raw, exposed, and vulnerable, but in a place for Christ to rebuild me. I would walk from my parked car to work feeling incredibly heavy, not knowing how on earth I was going to face seeing people, let alone be joyful for their pregnancies! I would ask the

Holy Spirit to lift my spirit, and by the time I walked through the hospital doors, I knew God's radiance was shining out of me because everyone smiled at me with such freshness.

We gave our whole-hearted commitment to the Cleansing Stream retreat. When asked to jump up and dance we were first on the dance floor, which was most unusual for me. I believed my intercessor would be given the power to heal me through Christ. The extraordinary thing was that intercessors were allocated randomly, but I stood before the same man four or five times. There were hundreds of us there that day. God was at work! It was so exciting. Coming away from the retreat I noticed I no longer had the back, hip, and long bone pain I'd had for two years and thought I'd inherited from my mother. I hadn't asked for prayer for this but I now grew quietly excited and expectant that God had healed my reproductive organs as well.

Sure enough, one menstrual month later I was pregnant with Emily. The scan at seven weeks was healthy. Praise God! So was the scan at twelve weeks. I couldn't contain my joy. I raved to the sonographer that God had healed me and removed the curse of freemasonry. Of course she thought I was a bit odd, but I was determined to declare God's victory at the first call. After that I'd only tell knowing Christians, and to others I would simply say it was a miracle.

Leading up to that twelve-week scan, I learned to savor my pregnancy as a secret between just God and me – and Andrew of course. It was like God made a covenant with me – my end of the deal was keeping my mouth shut. I thought this was probably to prevent me uttering any negative curse over myself while working in midwifery and around doctors where the medical language can be condemning. I grew to love and treasure this secret and felt determined not to break the bubble. It was a time for enjoying private intimacy with God – just Him and me.

I got through those twelve weeks where the world says a pregnancy is touch and go, by knowing that when I could tell the world it would be an incredible story. I couldn't wait to be able to tell my testimony at last. After the twelve-week scan, with some trepidation at revealing my secret, I broke out with the news to my eldest daughter. It was wonderful to tell her I was going to have a baby and that it was in here, pointing to my stomach. Her eyes grew wide with wonder and delight and she soon found a new peace. She said she knew "her children would now have an aunt or uncle." Such a generational thought for a then eight–year-old!

Emily was born at forty-one weeks, completely perfect and a perfect miracle. Thank you, my Daddy in heaven, my King of the Universe. One day a friend answered Andrew's question, "Why would God put a Christian through so much trauma when He has the power to intervene?" She simply said, as if straight from God's own mouth, "Because He didn't want your future generations tainted with the curses of freemasonry." God's plans are so much bigger and far-reaching than our own dreams. It's not just about us. It's about His future generations through us.

Looking back I remember feeling confused about what God wanted for my life, as we waited to get pregnant successfully for the seventh to twelfth times. I could see a number of avenues he might want me to work in but found it impossible to be decisive as I didn't know if a child was coming soon or not. It was the beginning of the year, and at that time the church home group we were leading was discussing what areas in the church we would volunteer our time to.

A dear friend suggested it was better to choose a specific avenue rather than work ones that were not my call. I found my solution in opening all doors, believing God would close them if they weren't where He wanted me to go. I carried on as a children's church small-group leader and leadership coach, and I helped facilitate a wonderful course looking at the root cause of emotional conditions, such as the cycle of addiction, hopelessness, shame, blaming, and punishing. I started working as a midwife again two days a week. I began the adoption application process and came off contraception. The only thing I stopped was ushering at church as it was difficult to stand for long periods during early pregnancies.

It was hard to separate the pain of the miscarriages from other painful trauma in my life to that date but God didn't need me to. I stood before Him broken open, my mess before Him, and He made my healing complete. I remember telling my counselor when I bumped into her after being blessed with Emily, that I felt there was nothing left to heal. It was all done. I'm not sure if that is correct in the eyes of God, but here and now I don't feel at all broken.

I believe the mentality of opening all doors and not being prescriptive to God over how he might bless me was key. He knew what was in my heart; I had prayed for children many times. After that, the ball was in God's court and all He expected of me was to keep faith and trust in His perfect timing.

It has been a very personalized journey with God as I expect it would be with anyone. I needed to ask God what it was He needed me to learn, do, think, and pray. That secret bubble I was in with God was where it all happened and where spiritual intimacy birthed a miracle.

A "NOT NORMAL" BLESSING

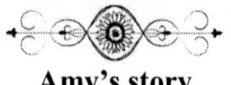

Amy's story

STARTING a family seemed like the most natural thing in the world for us. We got married young--I was nineteen, Mike was twenty-one, and never in a million years had we given a thought to not getting pregnant easily. In fact, we had never even spoken to anyone who had experienced problems conceiving.

We can still remember the day, almost five years into our marriage, when we started trying to conceive. I remember how much fun it was dreaming of our children to come. We would never have imagined that it would take another five years for our dream to become a reality. Natural conception? No, it would be anything but! If someone had told us back then that we would travel the lonely road of infertility right through to in vitro fertilization (IVF), we would never have believed them.

In the first year of trying we did our best not to worry. Yet every passing month increased our sense that somehow this wasn't going to happen easily for us. Up until this point life had been handed to us on a silver platter: marriage, jobs, ministry had all fallen into place. We hadn't encountered any real times of testing. We both started feeling we were facing a huge battle to have a family.

We had moved to a new city to take on the role as children's pastors at a church there. As the years passed by it felt increasingly ironic that we were children's pastors, then family ministry pastors without any children, without a family. Emotionally, this really took its toll and even made us question the role God had called us to. We never wanted the parents at church to think we didn't want children, so we decided to be open about our journey. Often we would feel inadequate. The pain of taking care of other people's children while not being able to have our own seemed unbearable, but we gathered a multitude of people who committed to pray for us.

My heart often broke, seeing how amazing Mike was with the children in our care and what a great dad he would be. It made us go deep into God's Word and hold on to His promises for us that we would indeed have a family one day.

We held tight to verses such as Psalm 113:9 (NIV), "He settles the barren woman in her home as a happy mother of children"; Exodus 23:26 (NIV), "… none will miscarry or be barren in your land. I will give you a full life span"; and Deuteronomy 7:13-14 (NIV), "He will love you and bless you and increase your numbers. He will bless the fruit of your womb…. You will be blessed more than any other people; none of your men or women will be childless, nor any of your livestock without young."

We continued to sow in faith but it was not without many tears. Mike would often find me lying awake crying in the middle of the night and really didn't know how to help me. Sometimes he would just wrap his arms around me and tell me everything was going to be okay. He found it very hard because like most men, he wanted to fix the problem but felt powerless to do so. Redecorating the church nursery was particularly painful for me, yet I clung to the hope that I would soon sit in one of those chairs nursing our own baby.

After trying unsuccessfully on our own for just over a year, we both undertook a string of fertility tests. I had a blood test on day twenty-one of my cycle over many months and an ultrasound. These both revealed I had polycystic ovaries and was not ovulating regularly – a condition that can but does not always affect fertility.

At the end of the second year we decided to go on three cycles of clomiphene (Clomid), a drug to stimulate ovulation, but this was unsuccessful. In December 2006, laparoscopic surgery revealed I had mild endometriosis behind my pelvis – a complete surprise. It was removed successfully. We thought pregnancy would happen quickly, but sadly, it didn't. Another three rounds of clomiphene later, our specialist decided that after three years it was time to refer us for publicly funded IVF treatment (which was available in the country we live in).

We had mixed emotions. Disappointment that nothing we tried had worked but relief and hope that we qualified for public funding. During 2007, while we waited, we gave clomiphene two more goes with a procedure called intrauterine insemination (IUI), which again was not successful. Clomiphene made my emotions very unstable. I cried all the time and was very irritable.

When these cycles failed it was devastating. A number of close friends got pregnant during this time, which was really hard to cope with. We were happy for them, but anyone who has traveled this journey knows that other people's joy just highlights your own pain.

We'd had enough of the drugs and procedures and we decided not to take any more until IVF. We were exhausted and our marriage needed a rest from the constant pressure treatment brings. Constantly focusing on trying to get pregnant was affecting every area of our lives. Making love just wasn't fun anymore. Getting pregnant was all we talked and breathed. We realized we needed to bring God back into focus. We did this by taking a long holiday to a ski town--Queenstown, New Zealand, not to try for a baby but just to have some "us" time. The beauty of the countryside spoke volumes into our hearts and we came away feeling so refreshed.

We began praying together again and started having date nights – something we had let go without really realizing it. We took turns planning something special once a week, which injected some romance and adventure back into our marriage. Once we did these things we found a great strength together to soldier on and our relationship today is much stronger for that time out.

We were still very unsure about IVF and grappled with God over doing it. Couldn't God just do this for us? Had we sinned? Were we lacking in faith? We often talked about these things, having learned by this stage that God didn't mind being asked the hard questions. He could handle it. He felt our pain.

Often well-meaning people implied we just needed more faith, needed to stop "trying," needed to get a pet, go on a holiday. Actually all we wanted people to say was, "I'm so sorry, this must be really tough." We needed people to pray for us, because there were times we had no energy left to pray at all. It became a constant daily choice to live in the land of hope and not disappointment, to go to where God was. This was especially difficult for me, as my emotions seemed to swing so much on the drugs. Counseling really made a difference, and I realized there was no shame in getting help, prayer, and wisdom at these times.

In June 2007 I had a prophesy over me saying God wanted to give us children but it would not be the "normal" way and that He would use our journey to bring life to many people. This gave me hope but also scared me, as I just wanted "normal." I didn't want to be the one who had to go through all the different fertility treatments to achieve our dream.

We were also approached with two private adoptions, which made us feel even more confused about God's path for us. We were, of course, open, and did wonder if this was part of our "not normal" journey. However, along the way we never stopped trusting God and listening to the leading of the Holy Spirit. We felt that before we considered adoption we were to continue along the path of fertility treatment until all avenues had been exhausted.

As pastors we had to face the ethical dilemmas associated with IVF. We feel strongly that life begins at conception and so each embryo has a right to live. The IVF drugs make the woman produce many eggs to increase the chance of fertilization, so we agreed we would use every frozen embryo we had, even if there were four, five, or nine!

We were booked for December 2007, but a few months prior we were asked to become assistants to a pastor who was very sick with cancer in another city. After much prayer and many tears we decided to postpone IVF and make the move. Mixing IVF with moving and a new job would have been unwise and way too stressful. The thought of yet another year rolling by without children was devastating, but we knew we were meant to go. This was confirmed when the pastor died six weeks after our arrival and we were handed the role of senior pastors. We wondered whether we had needed to take this step of faith and then our miracle would come.

After much prayer we decided to go ahead with IVF in late April 2008, so I reduced my hours to one day a week to eliminate as much stress as possible. I can still remember every injection, the nausea, and the emotional side effects. Mike was there encouraging me at most injections and it really felt like we were doing it together. I was proud of being able to administer the injections myself and even found the funny side of getting an early indication of what menopause would be like with headaches and hot flushes.

I found I needed to be kind to myself during the cycle and take time out for me. Something as simple as popping out to a café for coffee, going for a long walk, or getting a beauty treatment really helped. Some amazing friends were also there for us. They would make us laugh, let us talk about everything going on, or were fine if we just wanted to hang out and not talk at all. We were really specific with our prayer requests through each step of the IVF cycle and felt the prayers of friends and close family carried us through. We are so glad we didn't keep the IVF a secret and had this great support throughout.

I felt every emotion imaginable, often swinging from great hope to great doubt and fear. We clung to God like never before, believing that even though the success rate was only around 40-50%, we would be in that percentile. The two-week wait after our embryo transfer was the toughest and longest fortnight of our life, but on June 19, 2008 our dream finally became a reality when we found out we were finally parents. I had my first positive pregnancy test ever and have kept the stick to prove it!

On March 3, 2009, we gave birth to a precious baby girl conceived by IVF and the only embryo in our cycle to survive. She is a miracle – the embryologist called her the "beautiful one." We named her Rosie Grace, which means "God's gracious gift," after her great grandma Rosaly, one of the most beautiful people we know.

God has been so faithful to us and never let us go during our five-year journey. I continue to pray that He will never let us forget the pain of what it felt like to be waiting, so that we can comfort and help others in the same situation. Our story is summed up by our promise from God in Psalm 113:9 (NIV). Mike lovingly painted these words on the canvas hanging in our nursery: "He settles the barren woman in her home as a happy mother of children. Praise the LORD."

One year later …

It has been a year since I wrote our story down just before our Rosie Grace arrived into our world. She is the biggest blessing from God to us and every day I am so thankful that she is here, our miracle girl. Now, nine months later, I can't imagine our life without her. God has fulfilled the greatest desire of my heart to be a mother and I absolutely love it. She fills me with joy every day and I can't wait to get up each morning to look after her. However, in the last few months I have started to feel there is again more to come on our journey…we are not done yet. Rosie is beautiful, and although I wondered how I would get through the first few months of sleepless nights, reflux, and poor weight gain, by God's grace we have, and Rosie is a happy, healthy baby.

Since my period returned when Rosie was six months old, I have had an overwhelming desire to have another child. I really didn't think I would feel this so soon and am really afraid of what this might mean for us. I really don't want to go back to the emotional rollercoaster of trying again. However, I was reading our promise from God in Rosie's room and was struck by His word to us in Psalm 113:9 (NIV): *"He will settle the barren woman in her home as a happy mother of children. Praise the Lord."* There it was staring back at me...not "child" but "children." More than one. I have heard myself say many times to people since Rosie was born, "If all we can have is her, I will be so blessed." But honestly, I know if we couldn't have more children I would feel a sense of disappointment. I have always wanted at least three children, and yet if that doesn't happen I do not want to live my life offended at God.

One of the hardest things for me about our infertility journey has been that it has felt like the choice to have children or a certain number of children has been taken away from us. Recently I have had several friends share with me they are trying for their second or third child. I know it's never going to feel as heartbreaking as before to hear news of pregnancies, but I have experienced a few familiar ugly feelings.

I have felt a sense of frustration and "it's not fair," and even dare I say, jealousy, because I know it will probably happen relatively easy for these friends. For them it will probably only take a few months; for us, we have no idea how long it may take. In the five years we were trying I never once conceived naturally. We felt very strongly IVF was God's plan for us to have Rosie but not having any frozen embryos and having to pay for any future cycles really messes with my head as to whether we should do it again. I would love to think God would just do it naturally, and I have faith to believe He can, but if not, would we consider doing fertility treatment again? And when? I cannot answer this question yet and I am realizing that that is okay. This is all part of our faith journey, trusting in God each step of the way.

God is doing a healing work in me and I know there will be more healing to come. He has been speaking to me a lot out of Matthew 11:28-30 (MSG): "Are you tired? Worn out? Burned out on religion? Come to me. Get away with me and you'll recover your life. I'll show you how to take a real rest. Walk with me and work with me – watch how I do it. Learn the unforced rhythms of grace. I won't lay anything heavy or ill-fitting on you. Keep company with me and you'll learn how to live freely and lightly."

I have been very aware lately of just how tired and worn out I have been in all aspects of my life and especially in my walk with God. I am learning again to come to Jesus to find real rest for my soul. He is revealing to me His unforced rhythm of grace. What a beautiful thought that Jesus has an unforced rhythm of grace that is unique for each one of us. It is not harsh or ill-fitting--it's a new beat, a new way of life learned only in fresh encounters with Jesus.

We are not done in this journey of infertility and I am learning to be okay with that. I am learning to listen to the state of my heart. My heart was screaming in pain from our five-year season of unrelenting disappointment that had left me heartsick. This disappointment had, like a virus, infected every part of me without my really knowing it. The result, even when I was pregnant, was a numbness to life and to God. I am choosing not to ignore this, for out of the heart flow the issues of life. As I am waiting on God, He is breathing new hope into my life; hope for the future and hope for more children to come.

I once heard hope described as a "patient, confident expectation of good," and I believe hope in the goodness of God will be the key for me to walk out our journey in a way that will honor Him. This hope is for more than just us. God continues to bring couples across our path facing infertility issues. We are able to listen to them, encourage them, and pray with them with honesty and real empathy. I will choose to believe in the goodness of our God who can, as it says in Hosea 2:15 (NLT), *"transform (our) Valley of Trouble into a doorway of hope."* Just two Sundays ago a visiting preacher had a word for Mike and me that God has equipped us to see breakthrough because of our five-year journey to have Rosie. This word resonates in our hearts, and we are believing that God will use us and our story to bring life, healing, and breakthrough to many.

LESSONS ALONG THE WAY

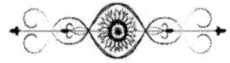

Samantha's Story

I stood in the queue at the pharmacy fighting back tears. I had to physically hold myself there as everything in me wanted to bolt out the door. It was so very wrong. I remember wondering how I had got there. How I had ended up being in a situation where I was about to purchase fertility drugs? Surely it wasn't God's plan for me. He was the God of abundance and promise and this was the very opposite of that. I had never felt so alone.

That was three years ago when the journey to try to have a baby was only beginning for us. It has been a rollercoaster ride of three cycles of clomiphene (Clomid), three cycles of IVF including a miscarriage, and month after month after month of hoping. When we started trying for a baby we were among the first of our friends and family to do so. Now we are almost the last couple in our circle without children.

I have always been an achiever – little Miss Get–It–Done. My belief was that if you applied yourself things would work out the way you planned. Life was well organised, and there was simply no room for failure. When something failed there was always a solution, you just had to look hard enough to find it.

Infertility blew that sweet little picture out of the water. It is something uncontrollable, a wild animal that bites and claws and hurts. There was absolutely nothing either my husband or I could do to make it happen. Of course there is the obvious, but that is not quite enough for us! My body is uncooperative to say the least.

A burst appendix when I was nine years old resulting in two rounds of invasive abdominal surgery and lots of internal scar tissue is problem number one. Problem number two is that I am not particularly fertile and my fertility has declined beyond my years. And to cap it off my body does not like drugs and reacts badly to all of them, so that's problem number three. Any one of these would be enough reason to seek fertility treatment but a hat trick of all three means having a baby is a huge challenge. One that God is more than up to, but a challenge all the same.

We started looking at the possibility of a family when I was thirty years old. Always career oriented, it took me this long to hand everything over to God and submit to Him in this area. I am South African. Sex education was not that comprehensive in the schooling system there, so timing was all guesswork for the first two years or so. When we realised that at some stage we should have got it right, we went to see a fertility clinic. The news was not good and continued to get worse with time and each passing experience. It was quite surreal. Every time we thought the news couldn't get worse, it did.

As we started down the fertility treatment route God spoke clearly to me about being strong and courageous. In Joshua 1 God tells Joshua three times to be strong and courageous before the end of verse 9. The origin of courage is from the Latin "cor" which means heart. For me it's always been about the heart. When I look back through my journals I can see God's handprint on our journey. That's reassuring for me because it's not an attack of the enemy or a generational curse but God's purpose for us right now.

"**Be strong and courageous**, for you are the one who will lead these people to possess all the land I swore to their ancestors I would give them. **Be strong and very courageous**. Be careful to obey all the instructions Moses gave you. Do not deviate from them, turning either to the right or to the left. Then you will be successful in everything you do. Study this Book of Instruction continually. Meditate on it day and night so you will be sure to obey everything written in it. Only then will you prosper and succeed in all you do. This is my command – **be strong and courageous**! Do not be afraid or discouraged. For the Lord your God is with you wherever you go" (Joshua 1: 6-9 NLT, emphasis mine).

I believe God's movement in our lives does not always give us the answer to our prayers in the way we think. I think God always hears and answers our prayers, but He may have something different to teach us or build in our lives than what we are expecting.

Often God has a bigger picture in mind; it's like we see the tree but He sees the whole forest. We were face to face with the tree and it was our whole perspective; we were so busy looking at that one tree we failed to see all the others.

* * *

It has been hard learning how to have hope in Hope and not in the hope that our prayer will be answered. My problem has never been not having enough faith that God will come through, but dealing with the disappointment if He doesn't come through in the way I thought He would.

After we did the obligatory three rounds of clomiphene (Clomid) to try and kick-start my body into producing eggs, a small series of miracles happened. Instead of having to wait a month to see the doctor, we got an appointment the following day. He then classified me as "severely infertile," a description I chose not to accept. He said our only option was IVF and referred us to the clinic's public funding coordinator. The wait for a publicly funded IVF cycle was a minimum of six months, but three days later we were told we could start as there was a gap in the program.

After the IVF cycle I fell pregnant. We were riding high on God's favor until December 22, 2005 when my nurse called to discuss my weekly blood test. I was six weeks pregnant. I remember her words exactly. When she asked if I was free to talk I replied that I couldn't talk in the open office but I could listen to her. She asked me to go somewhere so we could have a conversation. I somehow knew she was about to give me bad news. I was right; my hormone levels had dropped and miscarriage was a certainty.

I ran out of the office and picked my husband Michael up from work. I screamed at God in the car, "Why? How could you?" The pain was indescribable. We shut ourselves in our house and I lay in a foetal position on the bed with the curtains drawn. Even now it's hard to look back on the pain we felt. It was a physical pain like shards of glass being pressed into our hearts and it hurt to even breathe. I miscarried on Christmas Day 2005.

That was such a dark time for us and it caused us to question everything we knew or believed in. I thank God for friends and family who held us and saw that what we were feeling was just a season of grieving, because there were those who judged us. What helped immensely were those who were slow to judge. They looked at our circumstances and the season we were in. They saw our hearts instead of the muddle that sometimes came out of our mouths.

God spoke clearly to me in this season. He showed me a vision of a landscape ravaged by fire. In South Africa bushfires or veld fires are common each winter on the highveld area I grew up in. Winters are dry without much rain. It doesn't take much for a fire to start then rage across the tinder-dry veld, burning everything in its path. We used to drive along the motorways and see vast areas of blackened scorched land on either side of the road. God showed me that this is what had happened in my life. Everything had been burned up and all I could do was sit in the blackened, charred remains and wait for Him. I found this strangely comforting. Despite what had happened we were in His hand. He had this awful, terrible time under control.

The devastation of a veld fire is also miraculous. Not only destructive, the fires also bring new life. Plants stunted because other vegetation blocks their light and space start to grow with ease. Certain types of seeds and insects created to start growing only when activated by intense heat lie dormant in the soil waiting for a fire to pass overhead. God showed me that was what had happened. He had cleared the veld of all unnecessary growth and now the ground was ready. The intense heat had activated new things that would take root in me and grow. Over time I saw this happen as God built compassion, mercy, and trust into me.

Not long after the miscarriage God led me in my own personalised Bible study. It was incredible as He took me from one verse to the next. It was all about the heart, which was wonderful confirmation that He had us in his hands and we were on the right track.

He started with a favourite verse of mine from Proverbs: "Trust God from the bottom of your heart; don't try to figure out everything on your own" (Proverbs 3:5, MSG). Trust, courage, and strength are to do with the heart, and mine needed work.

As I read on to the next chapter, another old favorite was highlighted: "Above all else, guard your heart...for it is the wellspring of life" (Proverbs 4:23, NIV). I understood that the state of my heart dictated whether I lived life well, whether I would be strong and courageous, and trust God or not.

He then showed me yet another verse from Proverbs: "Fire tests the purity of silver and gold, but the Lord tests the heart" (Proverbs 17:3, NLT). I knew this journey was God ordained and he would test my heart again and again, as it is so important to every aspect of my life. If my heart is pure then I am pure.

He then led me to the last verse, which was both comforting and terrifying. "I have refined you, but not as silver is refined. Rather, I have refined you in the furnace of suffering" (Isaiah 48:10, NLT). Comforting, because again it showed me the purpose of what we were going through. We knew with our heads that everything God does has a purpose but sometimes that didn't quite get through to our hearts. I knew we were not through with the testing yet. Hearing from God so clearly gave me a sense of direction. I could not see a way through but I knew God could. All I had to do was try to stay with Him and trust Him.

We had our second cycle of publicly funded IVF a few months after the miscarriage. I knew early on that it had failed. I know almost immediately if I am pregnant because my body responds instantly. I took the pregnancy test early in the first round of IVF but even though I had no physical signs of pregnancy with the second cycle of IVF, we waited the obligatory fourteen days to find out. On the morning of the blood test I had a call with the news we expected. I was not pregnant.

I went to the toilet at work and stood in the cubicle fighting for balance. I had a choice about my reaction and God asked me to choose. It was almost like I could see myself moving through time to a door. I knew I would find grace and strength on the other side of that door but moving through it meant I had to submit and tell God what had happened was okay.

I moved through that door and found the strength to worship Him there and then. I saw myself dancing in the dragon's mouth and praising God. The enemy meant to bring me down in that moment but God lifted me up.

I call that ordinary door the "Door of Grace." I have noticed it's not there for long and can be found just after a crisis. If I choose to turn to Him and submit and worship Him in that moment, I have access to a treasure trove of strength and resources. The sad thing is though, I find if I miss that moment, it's really hard to get back there.

This sounds so holy when I look back and in a way it was, as God was in it. But in the middle was me, and I hurt… a lot. I am just an ordinary girl who is both sensitive and emotional. The last thing I would want to put across is that I had it all together and somehow sailed through this experience earning a heavenly brownie badge. I have learned a lot the hard way, through gritty, dirty, and exhausting everyday life. God has endured a lot of kicking, screaming, and the odd tantrum. He has loved me the same through it all and I am so grateful.

We waited for a year before trying IVF again. We used this time to wait on God and give him room to move. It was also a time for me to get healthy once more as IVF had taken a lot out of my body. It was a good year and we trusted God with everything we had.

When we felt the time was right we talked to the fertility doctor about another IVF cycle. He ran blood tests and the results were unexpected. My fertility had declined dramatically in the year since our second IVF cycle, so unless this third cycle was significantly better than the last two, IVF was no longer an option for us. We were devastated.

Although I had not responded well in the first two cycles of IVF, we thought we would just continue on until we got pregnant. I think in hindsight we had put too much faith in medicine, thinking that with medical science on our side, we could make this happen. The news from the doctor caused us to open up and ask people we knew to pray for us. We were desperate and cried out to God. I fasted for a couple of days and God gave us an amazing promise.

He showed me the passage from Exodus 14:13-15 and 17-18 (NLT) where the Israelites are between a rock and a hard place, literally! "But Moses told the people, 'Don't be afraid. Just stand still and watch the Lord rescue you today. The Egyptians you see today will never be seen again. The Lord himself will fight for you. Just stay calm.' Then the Lord said to Moses... 'My great glory will be displayed through Pharaoh and his troops, his chariots, and his charioteers. When my glory is displayed through them, all Egypt will see my glory and know that I am the Lord!'"

I knew all we had to do was stand and watch God go to war for us. God Himself would fight for us and the Egyptian (infertility) would never be seen again. This victory would be for His glory; winning was not up to my body. Relief flooded my whole being and I wept with gratitude. What an amazing God we serve!

Encouraged, we began IVF. I did not respond any better despite new and larger amounts of drugs, but the cycle was successful in terms of egg creation and I found myself in the familiar place of waiting to see if I was pregnant. Initially the signs were good and my body responded with the symptoms of pregnancy. But the day before the fourteen-day blood test was due, all the symptoms disappeared. I knew the test would be negative and it was.

How would we react? Well, we were exhausted and demoralised, to be honest, but chose to trust God. He had given us an amazing, clear promise and we held onto it. God is not a man that He should lie! If the promise was not for now, it would be for later. I won't lie to you, this was incredibly hard to accept. We had held onto the words He gave us with all we had. They were not for now. But again we had a choice: would we submit and trust or become bitter and twisted? No real choice, really. We chose to submit and trust.

* * *

We went on a long holiday, spending time relaxing and having fun together. After the IVF cycle we needed to reconnect and just be together. We arrived back in Auckland, NZ (our home city) to a question from someone we knew. A young girl was pregnant and six weeks away from birth. She wanted to give the baby up for adoption, would we be interested?

On wise advice we had been pursuing three options for a baby. The first was a miracle, the second was fertility treatment, and the third was adoption. The adoption assessment process was underway with the associated government agency, so this was a viable suggestion.

A member of the birth family met us in Starbucks. It was my thirty-sixth birthday. I remember the words she said to us: we had to accept that this baby was going to be ours.

I thank God we guarded our hearts. Something in us held back and the verse God gave us from Proverbs about guarding our heart held us in good stead.

The mother changed her mind a few days before the birth. It was really hard but not as hard as IVF. Still, we were really glad to say good bye to 2007 and start a new year. The last four months had been harder than anything we had ever gone through, but God sustained us and held us and lifted us up and beyond our circumstances.

A beautiful trait God has built in me is strength. Not a natural A-type personality strength, but strength that relies on and is built up in Him. I am an interior designer, working for a great company. Last year we won a project – a very particular project – a new design of *my* fertility clinic.

My boss asked if I could do it and initially I said no. As anyone who has been through fertility treatment will know, it's incredibly traumatic and the clinic represents that pain. Add to that the fact that all my treatments had failed, and I would rather have had a kick in the shins than walk through the door of the clinic.

But as I thought about it I began to see God in it. Who better to design the clinic than me? I could design it completely from a patient's perspective; I understand what patients feel and what they need. I prayed and knew I had to do it.

Was it hard? Incredibly. I was shaking the first couple of times I met with the clinic team. I then added fuel to the fire and underwent our third failed IVF cycle while designing the clinic. Insane?

In the natural, certainly. But with God I had the strength, and He graced me with the ability. I prayed really hard as I designed the space and it is perfect: all soft edges and warm tones, and it feels like an up-market house or hotel as the spaces flow into each other. I pray that the couples who come there trembling inside will find comfort and peace in the space. I declare that it's a place of breakthrough and hope and pray that couples who come in broken and torn will leave with their hearts' desire!

* * *

I was sick at home recently and watched the *Oprah Winfrey Show*. The theme was death; not a morbid look at death, but a celebration of life for those who are terminally ill. The show featured a young woman with terminal cancer who is living life to the absolute maximum.

She talked about perspective; how cancer has shifted her perspective on life. She looks on cancer as an odd kind of blessing, not a curse. She said life is about how you look at it. I was incredibly affected, particularly as she is doing all this without Christ. And the thing is that her "discovery" is biblical.

In the days that followed God began talking to me about shifting my perspective; about living life now, not looking back at yesterday or towards tomorrow. Why wasn't I living that way all the time? Well, infertility is a journey, and it can take a while to get from A to B.

I realised that, in order to reach B, my perspective had to change and shift to seeing where I am as a blessing and not a curse. It's about appreciating B because we receive so much there, but not always the physical answer to our prayers. The B place has such potential. The B place is where I am learning to live out the lessons God wants to teach me. The B place means freedom, peace, and joy. B is the rest God promises us. B is an incredibly beautiful place where I can see completion and fulfilment – my C place – in the distance, but appreciate where I am now, content to wait.

This B place helps me realise that my life is rich right here and now, free and unfettered by the wonderful demands of parenthood. It's bittersweet like a really good quality dark chocolate. It's rich and decadent, in the right way.

I am no closer to realising my dream of having children; I may even be further off than when I started but that's okay. I trust God will give me the desires of my heart in His prefect timing, and in the meantime, I love my abundant, blessed life **now**.

"But these things I plan won't happen right away. Slowly, steadily, surely, the time approaches when the vision will be fulfilled. If it seems slow, wait patiently, for it will surely take place. It will not be delayed" (Habakkuk 2:3, NLT).

Footnote

It's August 2009 and so much has happened since I wrote those words. We have walked through the deepest valley of our lives but also stood on the highest mountaintop. The constant through these times of testing and trusting has been my God. I am standing today because of Him. I cannot lift Him high enough. He is my strength.

Oh yes! Our mountaintop experience is a little boy! In November 2008 we adopted a little boy we named Reuben. Our "son of vision" arrived. Words are inadequate to describe the joy we feel at finally being parents, even ten months later. We love spending each day with Reuben and he is truly the apple of our eyes. We are continuing with fertility treatment and are nearing the close of that chapter, but that is a story for another day.

Please be encouraged! You are not alone on this journey. Stay close to God and He will give you strength. He is the source of what you need.

A SOVEREIGN GRACE RESTORES

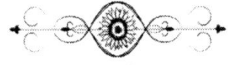

Lyn's Story
(as told to Catherine Sylvester)

I believe God promised us two kids, but as I got older I thought, "God, you may have promised, but please don't fulfill it." The more time passed, the more I felt I could not cope because of the age gap, purely the age gap. I couldn't be bothered getting up in the middle of the night. That was from forty-five onwards. That's twenty years of wanting. It's a long time.

When did you first feel there might be a problem?

I wanted four kids by the time I was thirty. Married at twenty-one, started trying at twenty-five, after two years it seemed there might be a problem. In my naivety I thought that after four years on the pill, it might be taking a while to get it out of my system. But two years should be long enough, shouldn't it?

During that time I was fairly chilled about it all and, being quite private, I wouldn't talk about it to anyone. It wasn't that I didn't feel I could, it was just our business and no one else's. When the family found out there was a problem, I was almost beside myself. I wouldn't talk to anyone. I wouldn't talk to my mum and dad. I wouldn't talk to my husband David's family. It was horrid. It was just so private and intimate.

So what made you seek assistance?

My mother encouraged me to seek help. With me being a fairly "hold it together, work it out, life goes on" sort of person, seeing me upset so often really worried her. "Let's get Lyn to a doctor," she said to David. She knew there was a problem and was concerned for my emotional state.

All I can remember about the conversation with the doctor, a Christian man, was that he said, "Job had his boils." How were Job and his boils going to help me have kids or feel better emotionally? I'm not sure I even understood what he meant. "Quite frankly, I know lots of people with many more problems than you have," he told me. I vowed and declared I would never go to him if I got sick!

From there I went to a gynecologist – a lovely man but not particularly helpful, as fertility problems weren't exactly his area of expertise. Time marched by without any real solutions to our problem, and eventually we found ourselves seeing a fertility specialist.

Were you affected spiritually as well as emotionally?

There were a few years between the "boil doctor" and seeing the specialist. I was so ticked off with that doctor. Not being able to have kids was totally consuming. It was like a reverse grief. Instead of time making it better, it made it worse.

I had terrible thoughts. I remember visiting a friend with her baby in hospital. As I held the little one I thought, "If I can't, she can't. I'll drop it." Isn't that awful? It only happened once, and I quickly stood over the bed. After that I stopped visiting mothers in hospital. I couldn't cope. I didn't, and still don't, go to baby showers. I could but I don't.

It was hard seeing women pregnant or with prams. I never thought about stealing a baby but my mother did. She confessed that when she saw a baby in a stroller and there was no mother

around, she would think, "I know someone who would love you."
It affected the whole family.

At that point God didn't have much bearing on our journey. My
thoughts were very clear: "Girls get pregnant all the time. God
knows we want a family." Any faith? No, it was just an expectation. To us it was more a physical issue than a spiritual issue.

*Were the specialists able to give a reason for your difficulty
conceiving?*

Our issue with getting pregnant was on David's side. We
weren't completely out of the game naturally, but assistance would
probably be required. It could happen but it was unlikely.

The specialist told us it would be ten years before IVF
technology would be specialised enough for our situation. Our only
option was a sperm donor. We were lined up on the waiting list but
when we got the call to say we were accepted, I just couldn't do it.
David would have gone along with my decision but I didn't have
peace.

I felt so uncomfortable; it really rocked my boat. There was no
way I could go ahead with it. It was all so new back then--you
couldn't seek wise advice or ask anyone, "What do you think?"

So when they rang to say our number was up and I said "please
take us off the list," the nurse thought I'd fallen off my perch. She
said she'd ring back in a few weeks, but my answer was still the
same. We have never regretted that decision.

*So where did you go after you opted out of the sperm donor
program?*

Even though we didn't talk about it much, people knew we
couldn't have kids. We were contacted about any baby that might
come up for adoption. "Would you like? Would you consider?
Would you like me to make enquiries?" I can't tell you how many
offers we had of a possible baby.

We went through social welfare. We went to their meetings
about adopting, did the paperwork, told them how many times we

changed our socks – all that sort of thing. But we felt a Christian had little hope of getting through. It might just have been the lady dealing with us, but it seemed that believing in God was unfavorable.

After filling out the papers we had a two-year window of opportunity to have a baby placed with us. People also continued coming to us with their "would you likes?"

In the first year the parents of a young girl living in the same city as my parents approached my mother. Their daughter was pregnant. Would we be interested in adopting the baby? We had lots of contact with Amy*, the birth mother, throughout her last six months of pregnancy. She even wanted me to have injections that would enable me to breastfeed the baby when it was born. She said she would let us know as soon as she went into labor so we could race down to the hospital to be there for the birth.

It was all very positive, and we didn't have a doubt that it was all on. We decked out the baby's room at our house and my sister spent ages sorting out baby gear.

Although we didn't make it for the birth, we weren't far off. I fed and looked after the baby in hospital for the first ten days of her life. We were even asked to name her. We chose Sarah Louise. Although it was a private arrangement, social welfare was on board and keen for us to be Sarah's parents.

Everything was in order. It was a done deal. This was our daughter; we were just waiting to take her home. I still have some of the feeding powder from the hospital. I haven't been able to throw it out. It's precious. It's a child, it's a memory.

That must've been an incredible experience. What happened when the time came to take her home?

David raced down at the weekend as he'd had to leave us to go to work. He even got off a speeding fine because the cop felt sorry for him.

I was about to go to the hospital to feed Sarah when social welfare phoned to say they wanted to come and see me. I told them they would have to wait, as I needed to get to Sarah, but they assured me the nurses would feed her and said they really had to talk to me then.

They told me it had all turned sour. Amy had changed her mind and the supposed father probably wasn't the father. There was another guy. It was all off. They apologized, as they'd had an inkling it wasn't going to work out earlier in the weekend. They felt they had let us down too. We told them we were so emotionally involved by then that had they told us, we wouldn't have been able to pull out anyway.

That must have been devastating.

We were broken. Absolutely broken. David's parents came down. My mother was broken too. I remember my father coming into the room and asking me to talk to her because she was so upset. But I was heartbroken and hopeless. My mother still says she has never experienced such grief. Not even when her mother died.

Though in deep pain, we didn't feel any animosity towards Amy. We felt God's grace in that although we were heartbroken, we weren't bitter. On the way out of town we stopped at a baby shop and bought a $50 outfit. That was quite a bit of money twenty years ago. We asked social welfare to give it to Amy for Sarah.

As we stood in the shop I can remember saying through tears, "I don't want it on the credit card. I don't want a reminder of what has happened." It was a finishing off; we loved her and this was something for her.

After that we stuck together and looked after ourselves. Everyone else had to work through their own grief.

And when you arrived home?

No one mentioned Sarah. It was a no-go for me for at least a year. It was a subject I was not prepared to talk about. My guard was up and I just wanted to get through it.

When we got home her room was back to normal: no evidence, which was very good. Everything was packed away. It wasn't until a year later that my sister asked what we would like to do with everything she had bought for Sarah.

How did it affect you and David as a couple?

As heartbreaking as it was to lose Sarah, I knew it wasn't going to destroy our relationship or us. All this fertility stuff can get ugly; your marriage can be hanging on by a thread.

David once asked me, years before Sarah, if I regretted marrying him. If I had married someone else I would've probably been able to have kids. It was lovely, because before we got married I had wondered whether it was right to marry him or was it just a good idea because our parents knew each other. God made it so clear that David was right for me. We should be joined in marriage and it was good.

I had confidence marrying David. If the package meant we couldn't have kids, it didn't mean our marriage was wrong. Because of that there was never any blame. When David asked me that question, and during every tough time on the journey, I was able to go back to that word from God and say, "No... we are supposed to be together." It was a defining time, where things turned around from ugly to nice. It was a wake-up call. It was wonderful.

For you, where was God in the midst of this?

Losing Sarah brought about a pivotal change in my relationship with God. It was the beginning of new beginnings. When we returned home without her, friends from church would say, "Well, did you pray about it?" I thought, "There's a novel idea." We hadn't prayed about it. We just assumed it was a God thing, an opportunity. Why wouldn't it be? Why wouldn't He want us to have kids? He'd promised us kids. Why couldn't this be it? So there hadn't been a thought that it wouldn't have been in God's plans or in His will.

I had started going to a women's group at church and discovered that they prayed and expected God was going to do something. And He did. That was a new experience for me. A new revelation.

As painful as our journey has sometimes been, without it my relationship with God might be quite different now. There have been so many moments I would not have known. They are so valuable.

I decided not to go through another opportunity for adoption without praying about it and knowing the answer. This was interesting, as not a month went by without people saying, "We have heard of... Are you interested...? Would you like..?" We were on a never-ending roller coaster ride of hope. "Is this it? Is it right?" It consumed us. You'd think it was helpful, but it was not. We had a big enough journey without this carrot we couldn't reach continually dangling in front of us. And the endless, "Should we? Are we prepared to go through this and be so vulnerable again?"

We didn't *not* consider adopting again, it was more a matter of seeking God on it. Years later we found out that a few months after Amy's change of mind, her mother told my mother that Amy had decided she'd made a mistake and was wondering if we would still be interested in adopting Sarah. Gratefully my mum said Amy was not allowed to contact us until after the paperwork was completed. We never heard anything. I was absolutely grateful mum made that decision.

How did people react? Did they understand the loss you had suffered?

When word got out about losing Sarah, I was mortified. I was so protective of this private hurt. I hated the fact that anyone knew. People didn't say much to us though. They were probably nervous or wondered if their comments would help or hinder us.

Our infertility affected the entire family. Immediately after my sisters had their babies was always a particularly difficult time for me… and my mother. She was split in two. She had one daughter desperately wanting children and struggling, and the other daughter having a baby. She wanted to celebrate yet felt bad doing so.

One day while driving down the road I was crying so much I felt there was no strength left in me to cry anymore. I felt desperately broken. I remembered something I had read in 1 Samuel 30:4-6 about when David had lost everything and they were about to stone him. He cried so much he had no strength left, but God gave him the strength to carry on.

Suddenly, as I recalled that verse, I felt peace – a real peace – like a physical warmth floating down from head to toe. It was amazing. I've never felt it before or since. But it was real and I knew I was in a safe place. It was like, "God, you understand me, you know I'm a mess but you love me."

Did that change the circumstance? No, but gosh, it was a defining moment on my journey. I knew God cared about me, loved me, understood me, and was for me. It was amazing.

So what happened next?

At least a year after Sarah and before the two-year window expired with social welfare, we were contacted yet again about adopting another baby. We felt healed emotionally and spiritually; we were moving forward.

Fay* was certain she wanted to adopt. Her son DJ would be ours. Still, this time I was a little more alert. I'd learned a few things and was a bit more guarded. I asked, "God, is this for us? Is this little one for us or not? You promised us kids. Is this part of it?" I felt strongly that God said no. I spoke to David about it.

Because we were so vulnerable and desperate to have children, we asked ourselves what if I hadn't heard correctly. We didn't want to live in the land of regrets. So we kept on walking; if the doors opened, then fine. But in my spirit I felt it was a no.

How was the relationship with the birth mother?

The relationship with Fay was less intense this time. We had less contact. When DJ was born we brought him home with us. We spent no time at the hospital as we had with Sarah.

The social welfare conditions required us to share-care DJ. Fay would travel to our home to spend a couple of days a week with DJ and us until seven lawyers and the courts finalized everything.

I was still very guarded. At the beginning I told Fay's mother it had to be the right decision for Fay. She'd made this commitment but if she changed her mind she had to do what was right for her and not worry about us. I wanted to release them. I needed to say it up front because I knew I'd get to a point where I couldn't.

The "no" was still on my mind. I had more of a caregiver's heart for DJ. It was like God protected my heart for me. I could care for DJ but it was different to Sarah--which turned out to be a very good thing.

We had DJ for six weeks, with Fay coming and going as things were shuffling through the courts. One day Fay's mother came with her. She thought I knew what was happening but I knew nothing. Fay had changed her mind, she couldn't go through with the adoption. She hadn't had the courage to say anything before arriving. She took DJ home then and there.

A second time! How crushing!

We were heartbroken. The next day, Sunday, not having slept until four in the morning, we arrived at church looking like we'd been through a washing machine agitator and wringer. We cried all the way through the service.

But then, another God moment. The preacher stopped mid-sentence and said, "Lyn and David, this is for you two. Know that God is able." It was another defining point for me. It was so releasing. God wouldn't even have had to get out of bed to make that decision change. He's so powerful. He sovereignly could've intervened if DJ was for us. I suddenly had absolute confidence that it was okay, because had God wanted us to have that little man we would have him. And that's that.

While we were sitting in the car after the service, an elder came up to us and said, "I want to pray for you." I was emotionally melting. We were going to lunch with relatives we could melt with, and here's this guy wanting to pray for us. In the end I said to David, "For goodness sake, if he wants to pray for us, let's get it over and done with so we can get out of here." So he did.

I will always connect that verse – the prayer of a righteous man has much power (James 5:16) – with this encounter. I cannot remember exactly what the elder prayed, but from that moment it was like all the grief lifted. We bought a gift and posted it to DJ.

Everyone else was upset. We were totally released. While discussing it on the way to lunch I asked, "David, how do you feel?" We both felt the grief had gone. God had supernaturally fast-tracked it. Amazing. We can testify to it because we had done the Sarah journey of so much heartbreak for so long, and here was this total, instantaneous release. So God.

People continued to approach us with adoption offers until I couldn't take it anymore and said, "God, enough. Please tell me. Will these kids you promised me come through adoption? I need to know." For a few weeks I sought Him. He'd tell me, then I'd say, "Not good enough. Tell me again." I wanted absolute clarity. I wanted to make sure I'd heard Him correctly.

The answer He gave me was from Jeremiah 33:14-15 (NIV): "I will fulfill the gracious promise I made … I will make a righteous Branch sprout from David's line." To me it was a no-brainer. If anyone rang, unless it was from David's family or David's connections, it was "no thank you." I'd just say, "Thank you for calling, thank you for caring, but no thank you." In fact, I actually took it to mean we would literally have children from David, but I was open to a bigger plan. Still definitely believing for a miracle, absolutely. Not a problem believing.

Life continued, and that roller coaster of every month wondering, "am I pregnant, am I not?" was exhausting. But God and I came to a bit of an arrangement when my period was two weeks late. I said, "God, if I'm not going to get pregnant, at least don't let my period come late again." And it never did. From then on it was always early or on time. Never that hope, that false hope, that maybe…

After DJ my mind and heart were settled about adoption. It wasn't for us. When people rang and said, "Would you be interested?" I thanked them with a no. David prayed too and came back with the same answer. We both felt peaceful about not pursuing any more adoptions.

How have the ensuing years been for you emotionally?

Through the years there have been many ups and downs. Despite knowing adoption was not for us, our desire for kids remained until our mid-forties. Then last year when I had an operation that meant conception would be impossible, I knew that was that.

Mother's Days were hard for such a long time. I recall writing a card for my mother, tears dripping onto the page. Once she spent Mother's Day with us. I thought I had coped wonderfully until she rang and said, "Remind me never to spend another Mother's Day with you!"

My pastor, a good friend, knew I was having a hard time and would pray for me without my knowledge. Afterwards she would ask how my day had been. Eventually I realized I'd sailed through it. She would also pray for me on days when someone's thoughtless comments had made a mess of me. By the end of the day the sun was shining again. I'm so grateful for the awesome power of prayer.

She helped me realize I didn't need to keep striving to achieve things myself. When I told her how hard it was to visit new mums in the hospital, she reminded me how God can change that. I felt I had a right not to have to do these things, but I can expect something else if I bring it to God. That was another pivotal thing – in the distress and the heartbreak God can actually change how I feel. I can walk victorious and free.

Although the shift from "please God now" to "not now God!" came for me in my mid forties, it didn't change the emotions of being broken or having that gap. Sometimes it still hits me – even recently and I am fifty-three now. Family photos are hard – everyone lines up with their kids, then there's just Lyn and David. When David's dad passed away recently, the other siblings' kids got a box of his stuff. We didn't have that.

My fortieth birthday was really hard. Another reminder, another milestone – no kids. Every year when people cried out "Happy New Year" I thought, what's happy about my year? I haven't got kids. Will next year be any different? It colored my life.

How do you feel about God seemingly not fulfilling his promise to you?

I remember someone asking me that very question. It's easy – they're His promises, His business. Yet just recently I read in Hebrews 11:39 (NIV), in the roll call of the saints, that they "were all commended for their faith, yet none of them received what had been promised." That really sealed and completed it for me. God is God. He's spoken and that's that.

Certainly for me, had we not been on this journey I wouldn't have found God the way I have. Finding the reality of Him makes a huge difference. And prayer changes things. Not necessarily the circumstances, but how you walk through them. You can walk through in a different way, with strength and confidence. Knowing He's there, He's with you, He's for you, and He is able. We might not have chosen it but God knows. He knows the beginning from the end. It's just a confidence, a trust that it's okay and we're okay.

To me, all you can do is go to the experts, the fertility clinic and the spiritual warfare people. Then you've done all you can do. Then you just walk. Do all you can and walk.

Finally, what has been the most important aspect of the journey for you?

I think to get a lot of the answers you've really got to hook in and hear God. A lot of people can say stuff to you. But the thing that holds it together is when you've heard from God. Personal revelation. That really glues it. When I talk about our journey now, it's the times when God intervened, or gave me clarity, or took away the grief, or gave me peace. Those are the defining moments. Those are the points I remember really, really clearly. All the rest fades as time goes by. But those pivotal defining times with God are so real. It's like it happened yesterday. Like signposts along the way. They're pretty precious.

*Some names have been changed

HOPE WITHIN THE WAIT

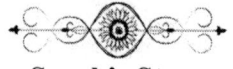

Sarah's Story

I never thought on that day when we were driving home from a weekend away, the decision for me to come off the pill and for us to start trying for a family would set the course for the hardest journey of my life to date.

This decision to try for a baby was supposed to lead us into a time of excitement and preparation, a joyous time as we expanded our family and created a little life together.

Instead I found myself on a journey of heartbreak: a journey of patience-testing of the extreme kind, of test results, and tears. Most surprisingly to me, a journey that would pull us back to church and change my relationship with God in a dramatic way.

Ultimately we were led on a journey towards IVF, the procedure I now hope will give us the child we desperately want.

We were ready. We had dated for a few years before we got married, had been married a while, done some travel. We were as ready as any couple can be for children. But our readiness meant nothing.

A year and a half of trying (on and off) and I knew in my gut something wasn't right. I was young, in good health, and had no reason to believe there would be any problem with conceiving. Our first step was to consult a natural fertility specialist. She recommended some tests and our results came in... low sperm count, low motility, and low chances of conceiving naturally.

We were assured it could still happen by working on our diets and making modifications. I look back now and think she was trying to be hopeful for us, but I think she probably knew we needed further help.

At that point we could have sat back and waited, tried modifying our diets, and given it six months to see if anything would happen. But after already trying for a year and a half, I'd had enough of waiting.

We decided to consult a local fertility clinic and were blessed with a fantastic specialist – one of the best. We were sent for ultrasounds and more blood and sperm tests to figure out the severity of our case. The results came in and all was not as we had hoped; they were worse than our original ones.

These results confirmed we needed treatment, and we were recommended for IVF. We were immediately put on the waitlist for treatment, a waitlist estimated at eighteen months... and this is where we currently sit, waiting.

With those results and our IVF "diagnosis" came feelings of shock. Even though we had known for some time something wasn't right, the reality of treatment and the wait ahead for it hit me hard. I literally felt numb for days. I remember crying in the shower those first few mornings and really struggling to see my way out.

My husband, whom I call the eternal optimist, really thought our second results would be better. He thought things would improve because he had worked on his diet and made some lifestyle changes. These new results shocked him too. I watched him struggle to grasp this new information and the fact that treatment was now really our only hope.

In those initial days I had difficulty accepting the reality that this was happening to us. This is just not how I thought things would go. Having such a long wait before getting treatment brought on a feeling of helplessness I'm not used to. We are months into our wait now and it is daunting still.

I struggle with the idea that getting pregnant and having children is something we are supposed to be able to do. I don't understand why this should be so hard for us! As human beings, isn't it a part of our purpose to reproduce, to bring forth the next generation? So why can't *we*? I struggle to make sense of it every single day.

In the weeks after our 'diagnosis' I was truly on an emotional roller-coaster. Every day I felt different. Some days I felt teary and upset and frustrated and helpless, other days I felt completely fine. These ups and downs are still happening, although a little less extreme most of the time.

I have days when I wonder if it's all worth it. Is it worth feeling like this? Should I just give up? My friends tell me children are wonderful and life changing but it's difficult to understand those feelings when you haven't experienced them. I have to trust maternal instinct and the knowledge we would make fantastic parents. I just hope we get the chance.

Shattered Dreams

I feel in many ways that my dreams have been shattered. I never thought about not having my own children, and a few of them at that. It never even occurred to me I might not. I think about the situation we are in and have to be realistic that there is a chance that it might not happen. There is a larger possibility we might only have one. That's hard for me to take. I am extremely close to my two siblings and I think about the impact they have had on me in so many positive ways. I feel sad that if we have a child he or she might never get that experience.

I feel like I've had to downgrade my dreams. That is truly how I feel. To get ONE child, ONE blessing would be amazing to me. To have the opportunity to raise even one of our own would be a huge blessing and one I would be so thankful for. Life has taken on a preciousness it never had and a fragility that never existed.

Hope

Sometimes it's a challenge being married to an optimist. It's not that I would class myself a pessimist; I generally see the glass half full. I'm just not quite at the level of optimism he's at most of the time. I'm a pragmatic type. I'm practical and I need a plan. I'm not completely without hope; its just hope tinged with realism. There have been a few times where we've been waiting for results and while he's busy preparing himself for better things this time, I'm bracing myself for worst-case scenario.

My theory is that if I can deal with worst-case scenario then I can deal with anything. It is a protection mechanism. It's about me taking myself to the worst place I can imagine, then I know I can deal with whatever eventuates.

I actually pray for more hope. I really wish hope came more naturally, rather than having to work on it as hard as I do. I love my husband's hopefulness. It's a desirable attribute and it really does keep me going.

Where Is God For Me?

I knew it would take something big to pull us back to church. We had both been out of church for a number of years, before we even started dating. We have many Christian friends and mix in mostly Christian circles. We just weren't going to church. It was not a priority. It wasn't something I even thought about on Sunday. We would often sit in bed planning our Sunday and church just wasn't part of it. Occasionally we discussed the idea of going back and had even tried to a few times, but just couldn't seem to get ourselves there.

Honestly, until recently, I still felt a little cynical about church; the organized nature of it. I didn't believe I needed it. We were too busy. We had enough friends. Our lives were too full for a church community – ha! God must have been chuckling away at my pathetic reasoning and excuses.

What's funny now is the times we discussed the probability of going back to church when we had children. Little did I know how ironic this was. It wasn't the way I thought it would be. It's the children we don't have that led us back!

I'd started to feel the call back to church a few months before our IVF diagnosis. It had been stirring in me for a while. We had talked about it a few times and I just couldn't shake it.

We are slowly progressing back to church. We've found a church home and are beginning to feel settled there which is great. I know God brought us back because He knows we need it. We still have a way to go…letting church life back into our regular life and allowing it to become part of our weekly existence. We still have to make room but I believe we will get there.

It was when I started to suspect things weren't going to happen for us that I felt God say quite clearly "You're going to need me soon." This sentence came to me more than once – "You're going to need me soon," and the feeling of "I'm not done with you yet." Then over and over in my mind I began getting this picture of a big thick rope as attached to an anchor, with God pulling at one end and us at the other. I could see His hands pulling the rope towards him. The picture is still so clear in my mind.

As I gradually began to let Him in, it was still hard to see His hand in all this. It was hard to see past my own emotions and blurry vision to get even a glimpse of His plan. But it happened in the shower one morning, only a week or so after we got our IVF verdict. I was crying, in a state of shock, and trying hard mentally to keep it together. My husband was away for the week and I had surrendered to my grief.

I felt God reveal something to me. I realized He had been placing some amazing people in my life slowly over the last few years, for this very time. One of these was Catherine Sylvester (Thursday's Babies), another was an old acquaintance I had reconnected with, who is my age and currently going through IVF treatment.

On that morning in the shower I realized many things had paved the way for me to give this the energy and time it needed. The fact I had been made redundant at my job earlier in the year and had recently started working for myself, removing the nine-to-five grind from my existence. The fact we had been placed with the best fertility doctor for our situation, the "fertility guru." It was that morning when I got a glimpse of His plan. I felt truly blown away and really felt like He was saying, "I'm not going to let you go."

It took the darkness of this situation to make a way for me to see the light. It took this confusion and frustration and heartbreak for me to really get it… He is ALWAYS there. I may not have realized it, I may have drifted away, but He hadn't given up.

He'd been waiting for me to whisper His name, to call out to Him. And He instantly responded. He's just waiting, the same as we are. Waiting for the knock, the phone call, the call up, ready to take His place at our side.

Reason

Although some things have become clearer, one thing I'm still struggling with is the reason for all this. Maybe it is what I've been talking about, to bring us into a closer relationship with God and back to church. But I believe there's more. I struggle with the reason and I feel quite desperate to find it. I frequently ask God to reveal it.

The fact that our specialist cannot give us a cause for the low sperm count and the fact that we have no history we can attribute to this occurring, makes me believe there is a purpose for what's happening to us. I have to believe that something really positive will occur as a result of this situation.

It's simply too hard to sit in this place without believing there will be a positive, healing, restorative outcome. Maybe writing this is part of that. Perhaps someone will be touched, someone will identify with our story. I hope so. I pray that the reason for all this will become clear. That's all I can do.

I have to believe God wouldn't give us something bigger than we can handle. He will use this experience, this time, to teach us, prepare us, and build strength within us. I know I am changing because of what we are going through. I feel in a constant state of change every day, and it's not such a bad thing. I'm reassessing many other things in my life because of where I'm at spiritually –

people I surround myself with, how I spend my time, my money, relationships. It feels like I'm going through an overhaul in every way.

One thing is certainly becoming clearer. All those times I walked away from Him and shelved Him, He never shelved me, never stopped trying to communicate with me – it just took something major for me to listen. Now I have to keep listening. I need to keep walking with Him and believe we will be okay, whatever the outcome.

"For I know the plans I have for you," declares the Lord, "plans to prosper you and not to harm you, plans to give you hope and a future." Jeremiah 29:11 (NIV).

AN INTRICATE PROCESS

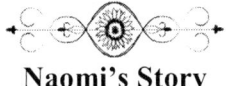

Naomi's Story

NOVEMBER 2002 and I remember the day like it was yesterday. We were going to try for a family!

Simon and I married young; I was nineteen, he was twenty-one. Nearly a year and a half later we made this big and exciting decision. I remember lying in bed thinking we could be pregnant right now! Little did I know our long journey had only just begun.

Sadly, that first month I got my period and the next month, and the next. I bought a secondhand cot that was on sale, some kids' books, and even nappies. I had no doubt that "next" month I would be pregnant.

Six months passed and by this time our friends had started getting married. Suddenly we'd been trying for a year. Our friends were getting pregnant but we weren't. Quickly in one sense, yet very slowly in another, three years passed. Throughout this time there was a lot of heartache. I thought, "It must be God's will, He has a plan, I must be patient, life is not about me, I'm okay and everything is fine." But deep down my true feelings were different.

I have always been the maternal type and practically the day after we got married people asked, "When are you going to have children?" This was so hard. I would always answer, "Sometime soon, I hope," not giving away too much. But after three years I was sick of being asked, and we started telling people it wasn't happening. This certainly stopped the inquiring! It was time to seek some medical assistance.

* * *

One of the hardest parts of this journey was the incredibly invasive tests the specialists gave us when we sought help. My hospital file is very thick. They presumed the problem was with me; Simon's only test showed his sperm were fine. It was time to seek some medical assistance.

* * *

Feeling the fault was mine was a heavy weight upon my shoulders until all the tests came back normal, which was fantastic. On the other hand there was still the looming question... why? I felt at times that it would've been easier if there *was* something wrong so it could be fixed.

I self-diagnosed endometriosis, thinking if it could be sorted out I would get pregnant. After surgery to check, it turned out I didn't have it at all, so there was nothing to fix.

After a painful operation, the doctors decided one of my fallopian tubes was blocked. Tears flowed - I felt so bad I couldn't provide a child for Simon and grandchildren for both our parents. Two weeks later they rang to say they had it all wrong; both my tubes were clean and healthy. Although excellent news, I only wished they'd got it right in the first place to save me that emotional pain.

To IVF or not

I had always said I wouldn't do IVF. I thought it would be "playing God." But as another year passed it became clear that IVF was our only option. How humbling. We thought and prayed for the next couple of years while we were on the waiting list. Thankfully my mother had advised us to put our name down anyway so that time would be ticking by.

We decided to go on an adventure holiday before making a final decision on IVF. A tour of Thailand that took us off the beaten trail to see the real culture was great for us as a couple. For years, although we tried not to let infertility rule our lives, we always thought about it and didn't really plan too much in advance just in case we got pregnant. We let our hair down and it was wonderful.

Two hours after a thirteen-hour flight during which neither of us slept, we arrived back home and went straight into five appointments with specialists. We sat there in disbelief. We didn't know how we'd got to this place and we didn't want to be there. We had still been having trouble fully deciding whether or not to go through with IVF. We had been praying, asking God to show us, but we didn't have any strong conviction about what to do. One option was IUI, where they inject sperm into the woman when she is ovulating, but we decided we had given that a good go on our own!

We didn't feel we absolutely shouldn't do IVF, so we decided to start the process, knowing that if we did change our minds, we just wouldn't start the drugs. Because it is possible to have two free IVF cycles in New Zealand (where we live), we knew that at any stage we could back out if we didn't feel it was right for us. The five appointments that day consisted of a counseling session, vaginal ultrasound, medical review, consent signing (which also explained the risks), and a nurse showing me how to inject the medications. The more we found out, the more we realized how much the drugs would affect my system. We left the clinic feeling overwhelmed and hoping we were making the right decision. On the trip home both of us were reflective but starting to get excited by the prospect of possibly getting pregnant. However one thing we have learned over this time is that we cannot always expect to get what we want. We must always trust and hope in the plan God has for our lives.

A diary entry for this time reads, "The last five weeks have been overwhelming. The thought that we are actually doing this is kind of scary and unbelievable. But I have been working through the issues and I'm starting to feel better about going through the process. The injections, moods, and emotions are playing on my mind but we have to hope we are doing the right thing. It has been hard knowing what to do but this is the only open door so far!"

The drugs begin

The process started on day one of my cycle, April 11, 2008. I was to go back on the contraceptive pill to ensure my cycle was full and normal. I started feeling sick, extremely tired, and had sore breasts. My next period arrived in early May, a blood test on day three set the rest of the dates for the month.

On day twenty-one my drug kit turned up: a black bag filled with about sixty-five needles and hormone drugs for the month. This was one scary bag, but I eventually got used to it all. I had a week to read up on everything and get familiar with how to inject myself. The first drug, Buserelin, basically shut down my system and put me in a menopausal state. It was weird to be going through menopause at the same time as my mother, although it was nice to relate and sympathise with her.

By this stage I had endured seventy-eight unwelcome periods. Just before Simon left for work, I got the needle out and wiped my tummy and the bottle with a special sterile pad. I loaded the needle with the Buserelin and sat there pointing it at my tummy. I didn't want to do it but I didn't know why. Simon suggested I look at him and put it in. Nice idea but I would rather know where I was putting that needle! Simon was wonderful and patient with me. He knew how hard this was and I just needed a bit more time to get my head around it. We were finally starting!

IVF can be hard for men too as there is not much they can do except watch their wives have countless blood tests, operations, internal examinations, and ultrasounds, then stick needles in themselves and totally manipulate their own system. Having a supportive, loving, caring, patient husband was amazing.

We were on the way. Simon gave me a big hug and took off to work. My dad phoned too, which meant the world to me. Our parents, extended family, and friends had all been so supportive while we were making our decision. Knowing they cared so much made this easier to cope with; we were so grateful.

My brother-in-law Stuart sent me a text saying, "This is my command – be strong and courageous! Do not be afraid or discouraged. For the Lord your God is with you wherever you go" (Joshua 1:9, NLT). He hadn't known how much I was struggling that day. How like God to give me the promise I needed at the right time.

The previous day some Christian friends had been judgmental about us going through with IVF. This broke my heart and made me feel like the worst sinner around. I was shocked they would say such things. I had finally come to the idea that maybe it was okay to do IVF but after that night I felt miserable. The verse in Stuart's text really helped me through that awful time. Words hurt people. Another lesson we have learned is not to comment on difficult issues or give an opinion unless we are asked and definitely know what we are talking about.

That same day some friends sent us an e-mail saying they had prayed for us and felt they should tell us, "The Lord wants to give you joy. His light chases away the darkness. No more fear. He wants you to know that you have His love and His favor. He's not angry with you. He loves you so much. Believe in Him, He is the truth". Once again God worked through people to help us in a time of need.

After starting the second stage drugs called Gonal F, the clinic monitored my progress every two days. The drug stimulated my ovaries and made extra eggs, as normally we make one a month.

We arrived at the clinic with butterflies. After all this time it came down to the next two weeks. Every second day I had a blood test and an internal ultrasound. The test showed I had three healthy follicles on one side and eight on the other. I had to return a few days later because they hadn't grown much.

The following night I was alone and had trouble injecting myself. This was the first time my emotions got the better of me. I lay down and had a big cry. I was disappointed at the outcome so far, worried that it wasn't going to work and sick of all the injections – I had done about fifty and was sore and bloated.

Two days later I was ready for the egg retrieval. By then I had five on one side and thirteen on the other. That night I injected the final drug called ovidrel, which makes the egg come away from the side of the follicle, ready to be picked up. The appointment was set for Friday at ten a.m., so at ten p.m. on Wednesday I had to do the injection. The timing is critical here – it must be thirty-six hours before pickup. If you do it too early or too late the egg will either not be ready or have already left the body. Such precision!

It was wonderful knowing that was the last injection...or so I thought.

Egg retrieval

Friday morning, June 27, 2008 finally came. I remember being excited. Things were looking good and I was so pleased we were nearly finished. Just the operation to collect my eggs and we'd be done. I changed into my fancy gown and was given a sedative. They also put in a line for pain relief. One of the doctors came to explain what would happen. They would go internally and pierce through the uterus to the ovaries then pop a needle into each follicle. A pump operated by the surgeon's foot sucks out the fluid and inside that should be an egg, but that's not always guaranteed. The tube is then passed to a scientist who examines the eggs under a microscope and gives everyone an update.

I woke up after two hours to a bunch of beautiful pink tulips from Simon. The nurses came in with the biggest muffin I had ever seen and a delicious hot chocolate. They had retrieved fifteen eggs! Wow, that was amazing. Getting eight is really good, and I almost doubled it. I felt awesome! Thank you Lord, I prayed. We needed to feel this was what we should be doing, and this seemed like confirmation to us.

Simon had given his sample earlier. The good and bad sperm are washed and separated. They put each egg in a little dish, add fifty thousand sperm, and leave them in an incubator overnight to do their thing. Simon said the lights were dim and romantic music was playing.

I wasn't able to sleep that night, so much was buzzing around in my head. Simon's aunty and uncle arrived when we were all in bed so I got up to welcome them. It was going to be a great family weekend. On Saturday morning we were all catching up and having a wonderful time while we waited for a call from the clinic to let us know how many eggs had fertilized. I had been saying I would be happy with one but the likelihood was at least seven or eight.

The phone rang, "Naomi, it's Aloma from the fertility clinic." Something in her voice worried me. "Naomi I don't know how to say this…" My heart sank. "None of the fifteen eggs fertilized, I'm so sorry." Time just froze. It was a really weird feeling. She continued, "I'm sorry, honey. We are all shocked here. This doesn't happen very often, and with your amount of eggs we were expecting a good return."

I was stunned, numb. I put the phone down, looked into Simon's eyes, and said, "None of them worked." I burst into tears. All hope drained from my body.

I felt embarrassed, empty. It was as though all my babies had died. My thinking was, "Why? Are we doing the wrong thing? Maybe God doesn't want us doing this. I'm so tired of making decisions and now we have to make more of them. How do we face family and friends when we have failed again? How disappointing, all those drugs and injections for nothing." It was simply awful. Simon's mum came and held us while we cried. She was really wonderful and prayed with us.

When I rang my parents my poor dad answered the phone. He was shocked. I was beside myself and embarrassed that I couldn't control my emotions. He passed me quickly onto Mum, who didn't know what to say either. There wasn't much she could say. It was so hard telling everyone it hadn't worked. I'm not normally an overly emotional person but with so much hope and hormones running through my veins, I just couldn't control the tears.

Simon's grandmother dropped to her knees as I was kneeling on the floor. She wrapped her arms around me and held me so tight. I was trying hard to pull myself together but it didn't last long. Surely there were no more tears left. She had struggled to get pregnant herself and knew the pain I was in. She is a wonderful, godly woman whom we admire so much, and to have her pray was very calming.

By eight thirty that night I was exhausted and still feeling down but trying hard not to let it ruin the lovely family weekend. I wanted to hide away in a cupboard. In bed that night Simon and I finally had a chance to talk. It was a busy household with eight people staying. I felt he had been hiding his emotions by being jovial. It was hard seeing him getting on and laughing and joking with people all day when I was feeling so awful. Of course he was shattered, but knew he needed to be my strength and try and keep positive. The hardest day we had ever been through finally came to an end and we slept.

What is the next step?

A couple of days later we were in the clinic, ready to find out what would happen next. I was determined not to cry. Would they consider us again? How long would we have to wait? Did we want to do it again? Was it the right thing to do? We prayed, "Lord please help us, we are so confused."

The doctor reiterated that they were all shocked and sad for us, then gave us some incredible news. They had discovered why we had not been able to get pregnant all these years – our eggs and sperm would not bind. We finally had a reason! It was amazing to know that through no fault of our own that we were having difficulties.

It was daunting to realize I would have to go through all that treatment again, but this time they would take one egg and inject one sperm into it to guarantee fertilization. We could still face the same outcome as the last treatment, but our odds were better. God is in control and His will prevails. We learned to accept that truth in times of pain. We couldn't lose anything more and had everything to gain.

We came away from the appointment feeling a lot better and ready to face the world again but we were both emotionally drained. Mum was in our kitchen cooking us dinner when we arrived home. I ran in and burst into tears. I just needed a hug from her. It had been a hard two weeks and it was so nice to be home. Many people visited over the next few days with flowers, gifts, chocolates, and cool pictures their children had drawn. It was so lovely but hard to face people too. We were surrounded by wonderful, understanding, and loving family and friends. Praise God.

* * *

We started the second cycle of IVF on Tuesday, August 12, 2008. The first round of drugs went well, but I felt worse than the previous time. After the second drug on Sunday, August 24, I reacted very fast and felt quite unwell, extremely tired, and sore in my tummy.

Eventually we met with the specialist and discovered I had twelve follicles on one ovary and fourteen on the other. No wonder I wasn't feeling well. The last time there were only eleven in total. The follicles still needed to grow a bit. Over the weekend I continued to feel awful while my stomach kept expanding. I looked pregnant! The pressure in my stomach was so bad.

The scan revealed that I was very ready to lay some eggs. They retrieved twenty-four–an amazing amount, considering eight is about normal. Being an egg-laying machine is great except that I got hyper stimulation and remained very unwell. It took a long time to bounce back to normal. We ended up with twenty embryos. This was a huge amount, considering we lost all of them last cycle. We had hope and confirmation again.

Monday, September 8, transplant time, was a strange and exciting day. They told us the procedure and showed us the embryo up on the screen. It was unbelievable. God is so powerful and amazing. To see an embryo, our embryo, was surreal! I lay on a bed, they slipped in a long tube with our little embryo in it, and after five minutes they said, "You are free to go."

I couldn't believe I was allowed to move and go about my day as usual. Of course I was still extremely tired, in pain, and needed rest, but there was an embryo inside me. It took a few hours before I thought it was safe to go to the bathroom, even though I really knew this wouldn't affect anything.

Then the dreaded wait to see if the embryo had taken. The longest two weeks of our lives and to top it off we both got the flu. I needed to take one more drug at this stage and the side effects were not pleasant: terrible stomach cramps, nausea, sore breasts, and more general physical misery than with the other drugs. I wasn't a pretty sight.

So many thoughts and emotions were flying around. It consumed my thoughts; knowing I had an embryo inside me and could be pregnant, but at the same time I didn't want to get my hopes up. I did whatever I could to distract myself and keep busy.

On Wednesday, September 17, I started getting massive back pain and lots of cramps, mainly from the drugs I had to take for up to seven weeks if I fell pregnant. I thought, "That's it, it hasn't worked, I can't get pregnant."

On Friday when I went for the first of two blood tests to find out what had happened, I told the nurse there was no way I could be pregnant. I felt premenstrual, in more pain than I had ever experienced before, and I had been on painkillers for the last two weeks.

Saturday came and I had a little spotting. We were devastated. If this embryo didn't take, we would have to wait six months before trying again because the clinic had run out of funding for the year. Six months seemed a long time after six years of trying to get pregnant.

Simon's mum rung and we told her it hadn't worked. We still had to wait for the results that afternoon, but we knew. We had planned a day at the beach and decided to go anyway. Simon was waxing up his hand-made wooden surfboard when my cell phone rang at 1 pm. It was Katrina from the clinic. I wasn't expecting the call for another few hours.

"You're pregnant!" she said.

"What? I can't be. I bled this morning!" I replied in shock.

She continued, "That's normal. You are very pregnant. Your hormone reading should be 100 and you are 340."

Life just stopped. I couldn't believe what I had heard. I hung up and shouted, "I'm pregnant!" We had a big stunned hug but it didn't seem real. I couldn't think straight and didn't know what to do with myself.

I immediately phoned our parents and my brother and sister. It was crazy telling them. I could finally say, "Mum, I'm pregnant!"

A couple of days later and I was nearly going crazy waiting until the afternoon to find out whether my next blood test showed my hormone levels had risen enough for me to be still pregnant. We had been on the biggest roller coaster of our lives and it was still going. "You are most certainly pregnant, Naomi! Your levels should have doubled to around 600 and you are 1296! Congratulations, we will see you in a few weeks for a scan." So it was true, I was pregnant! It seemed surreal. We had the most amazing couple of days celebrating and sharing with family and friends.

By Saturday I freaked out a bit, because it was still so early and I didn't know if I could hold a baby. I became quite scared but prayed the Lord would hold us in His arms.

Within days the morning sickness started and it was awful. But I was very happy. The backache and cramps up to eleven weeks were very disconcerting. Each ache, pain, and cramp made me wonder if I was going to lose this baby. I didn't want to be pessimistic, and from the outside I looked confident and loved every moment. But on the inside I was holding back and didn't really feel like I was trusting God. It was a strange place to be.

We had the first scan at seven weeks. And there it was. A tiny little flutter. Our baby's heart. My official due date was my dad's birthday, May 27, 2009.

It is so hard to explain the feelings following this appointment. We were really pregnant. After six and a half very long years, there was life inside me.

At ten weeks I started to bleed. I was shocked. I took off to my midwife and there was still a heartbeat. Oh, the relief. I kept reminding myself that God is in control. A couple of weeks later more bleeding meant we had an emergency scan, but thankfully, everything was okay. It was hard work emotionally. I bled again at sixteen weeks and then at eighteen. By this time my mind was going nuts. I desperately didn't want to lose this baby but knew there was nothing I could do if that was the case.

The scan showed that my placenta was previa, meaning it was over my cervix. It was more than likely I would have to have a caesarean. That was fine with me and it explained the bleeding. From then on I wasn't allowed to clean, hang washing, go for walks or have sex. By twenty-eight weeks I started to feel that maybe we were going to have a baby but after everything we'd been through, I was still nervous.

My placenta didn't move, so we booked Wednesday, May 20 for the cesarean. This was wonderful. A lot of people thought I would be disappointed at not giving birth naturally, but our whole process was unnatural so it didn't matter to me. We had everything ready, people wished us well, and we were off. Both of us were able to stay in the hospital. On the drive there the thought that in an hour we would be parents was overwhelming. It was the last part of this journey and a new one was about to start. As I heard my baby cry for the first time, my eyes filled with tears After all these years of waiting God had blessed us with a child.

A boy! We had a son. We named him Reuben Thomas. Baby Reuben was finally in my arms. I just couldn't get my head around it. I was a mother to this beautiful little boy. Simon then cuddled with us and we had our first family photo.

"He is alive and well. Lord, thank you for answering my prayers again. You have been so faithful to us. Thank you for this amazing gift. You never change, but you have changed us."

We are truly blessed to have gone through this journey and ended with an amazing son, and even more to be a part of this book and share our story.

The lessons we have learned are to trust God fully with everything. His timing is perfect. He will open and close doors as He sees fit. We had to trust His way is for good. We also learned not to judge others or give our opinion if we don't know what we are talking about.

We believe God has used this journey so we can reach others. Over the past two years we have become great friends with many people in the same situation. It is wonderful to pass on our knowledge and share why we were able to get through this. We struggled, but it made it easier, knowing that God had His plan, and was working it out for our good and His glory.

LIFE THROUGH THE LOSS

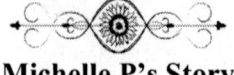

Michelle P's Story

April 16, 2007

I birthed our wee one at home on the night of April 14. I was meant to be just over sixteen weeks pregnant. The ultrasound scan four days earlier had shown a perfectly formed baby measuring only eleven weeks and two days old, with no heartbeat detected.

The beginning of the end…

It was a lovely Easter Sunday afternoon and we were in the company of friends, when somewhere between four and five p.m., I went to the toilet and found bloodstains on my underwear. My heart sank for a moment. My midwife had been unable to find a heartbeat at twelve and fourteen weeks, but we were both confident that the pregnancy was okay, as I had no history of miscarriage and two hassle-free pregnancies both ending in my two eldest boys being carried to full term and birthed naturally. I was therefore happy to go back at sixteen weeks to listen for the heartbeat.

My husband Craig and I brought our concerns and anxiety before God and submitted them to Him in prayer. The day before Easter we had read a woman's account of her remarkable pregnancy with her fifth child. That story, as well as our unfailing belief in a God who is able to do the impossible, inspired hope in our hearts for a miracle.

On Monday night I had severe tummy ache, which resulted in a bout of diarrhea. I remember thinking I would get a scan the next day to determine the cause of the bleeding. So that's what we did, and the scan did not show what we had hoped for.

Still it did not feel like the end. We did not deny what we saw and agreed with the prognosis, but we just could not dismiss the fact that God is able to do immeasurably more than what we ask or imagine. So we did what we knew we had to do and that was to act on our convictions. We declined the offer of a D and C, choosing to wait for either a natural miscarriage or a miracle story to share. We fought and fought for the latter. Craig fasted from food and I fasted from computer use and chocolate consumption as we sought God in prayer.

The days ticked by, the bleeding stayed much the same. We remained hopeful, with lapsed moments of feeling like giving up. We felt the support and prayers of those standing with us, believing with us for the miracle of miracles.

I woke up on Saturday with no discomfort, but by late afternoon I felt a constant cramping. By six p.m. it was reaching close to my low–pain-tolerance level. I remember looking at the clock at eight forty-five p.m. on yet another trip to the toilet, then shortly after out came the fetus. I carefully laid my baby in a container and found myself thinking, "You're beautiful baby. Mummy never gave up on you."

To summarize the rest of the story, I stayed nil by mouth overnight at the hospital, waiting for a scan and then waiting some more for the doctor to tell me whether he thought I needed a D and C. I was finally discharged at four p.m., no D and C needed, and no blood transfusion needed though my hemoglobin count was low at ninety-one.

And so it was, we have no miracle story to tell.

For reasons unknown to us while on earth, God chose not to answer our prayers as we intended Him to. Our baby boy (I'd asked a nurse or doctor at the hospital to look at the fetus to see if she could determine the gender) is now with Jesus. We look forward to the day we will meet him in heaven.

And so the fasting is over; time to eat and praise God for a lot more. Sorrow we'll feel, probably at the most inconvenient times, so if you're around when it strikes, a hug will comfort much.

A new chapter begins…

It's been four days. Mostly I have been in good spirits. But there are questions and thoughts; all evidence that I am wanting an answer.

Was it something I did? Was it the time I handled an artifact at my sister-in-law's house (she's a feng shui master)? Was it the day I lost it at Samuel, the eldest of my two sons? Did I go into any place filled with spiritual dark forces?

I am comforted by the knowledge that this baby boy has eternal life with Jesus. However that begets a whole new set of questions. Why would I want to bring forth another child if potentially, as a grown up, they may choose not to have a relationship with Christ, and therefore if they die rejecting God in their life, then they will be eternally separated from God? I guess my justification is that they could just as well choose to live their life for God, as a result of which many would be touched or influenced to have a relationship with Christ.

Some people would say all things happen for a reason. Craig and I do not necessarily agree with this sentiment. I don't think it's God's will for a baby to die. Bad things happen, but they're not necessarily part of God's plan. Certainly, though, God can use the situations and experiences for good.

April 19, 2007

Tonight as we were having dinner Samuel said, "Our little baby brother is with Jesus." We asked him what name we should call baby brother. He said Rebekah, bless him. After we explained that's a girl's name, and that we really should have a boy's name for our baby brother, he came up with Zac. Craig and I felt a sense of unity in that. And it's rather appropriate meaning: "The Lord remembers." Out of the mouths of babes…

April 20, 2007

Emotional triggers are so random. Most of the time I'm fine, happy even – ah my two active boys bring much joy to my heart, and as for my loving husband, he's just the best.

But as I stood next to an obviously pregnant woman today, I was suddenly filled with tears of loss. Boy, was I feeling sorry for myself for having lost the knowing that I was soon to have a proud preggy tummy to show off and rub. Seeing that tiny baby asleep in the sling on her mummy standing opposite me – man, I was looking forward to doing that in September/October. Sigh…

Oh and what about the incident when an acquaintance innocently asked, as you do in general small talk, "So are you stopping at two?" I felt awkward for her when I, being the bare-all type of person I can be, told her what had happened. I don't know if she felt she might have been insensitive, but really she wasn't. How could she have known? Perhaps I should have just said something like "we're working on more."

April 22, 2007

What broke the dam so tears flowed and flowed silently this morning? At church during worship we sang "I Stand in Awe of You" by Mark Altrogge. It contains the line, "Who can grasp your infinite wisdom?"

Not I, Lord, not I. Who can grasp your infinite wisdom? Not I.

April 24, 2007

Beautiful quote:

"Sometimes love is for a lifetime. Sometimes love is for a moment. Sometimes a moment is a lifetime." (Martin Luther King)

It has so much depth in meaning for me now.

May 2, 2007

In the past few days I have read or heard stories of people having multiple miscarriages. Like yesterday when a friend told me about a lady who had three miscarriages after her third child was born. I feel so bad because while I understand their pain and loss, I can't help turning it into an "about me" thing. I was thinking/praying, "Let that not be my cup, Lord!"

May 3, 2007

Tonight Craig asked me what I'd like for Mother's Day. I had not anticipated how that question would affect me – it broke the dam of tears again. All I could think of in response was, "Baby Zac."

May 4, 2007

I have been having major cramps these last few days. Initially they were mild during the day but more pronounced at night. The last two days the cramping has been constant and painful enough that I need to lie down. I have even contemplated taking painkillers. I finally did this afternoon – and boy, that one tablet made a world of a difference!

Do I need to be concerned?? Part of me thinks this must be good, as it means my body is expelling the remaining things that shouldn't be there. Part of me wonders about the possibility of having to have a D and C after all. Today I got the results of the blood test taken two days ago – HCG level is down to 3.0 (it was 5.0 a week ago). I asked the nurse about this cramping business – she doesn't seem too concerned but said to see the doctor if I feel dissatisfied after the weekend.

May 6, 2007

The sermon at church this morning was about the rich young man and the challenge that comes with that story. What in my life am I holding on to that is hindering me spiritually? Anyway, it got me off on a tangent, thinking about my desire for a family with four living kids. We would welcome more if God chooses to bless us so, but for some reason I'd like a "large" family of four kids. It got me wondering if my desire for this could turn into an idol in my life. I wondered if I actually idolized the picture perfect family of mum, dad and four kids.

We also sang a Vineyard song by Marc James, "Surrender." I vaguely remember having sung it before, but this morning it brought tears as I sang those words in a different light, I'm sure, than the writer's intention. I realized I had to lay down my dreams, my rights, and give Him my heart fully.

It made me think of my dreams for my unborn baby Zac; my right to have been able to carry the pregnancy through to birth; my pride to be able to say God's favor is upon me as I have never suffered a miscarriage; the promise of new life – my next pregnancy.

May 24, 2007

It is my mandate to never give up. If God says to be fruitful and multiply, and if it says in the Bible that children are blessings from God, then it is easy to conclude that the desire to have children is from God and it is a good desire to have. It is also easy after suffering a miscarriage to think fearfully, "I don't want to go through that again" or "what if it happens again?" I choose not to bow down to fear.

We lost Zac, but one day we will be reunited in heaven. To have another baby will never replace our beautiful boy who lives in our hearts.

I know what lies ahead of me – that no doubt I will be assailed with all sorts of fearful imaginings through the next pregnancy. But God will walk through with me, and I will look fear in the face because my God is the God of impossible and the victory is in Him.

Ten months later…

Friday, March 14, 2008

Twelve weeks, two days along. Uncharacteristically, but understandably, we decided to have a nuchal fold scan, as I really wanted to see the heartbeat for reassurance. The scan indeed showed a healthy baby with a strong heartbeat. The results also showed a very low-risk pregnancy. Praise God, all glory to Him.

Monday, March 31, 2008

Fourteen weeks, five days along in the pregnancy. Had a routine mid-wife's appointment. When the midwife tried to listen for the heartbeat, she found nothing. As I lay on the bed I had a sinking, all too familiar feeling – is this déjà vu? Part of me rose up and dismissed this as a scare tactic from the enemy. "I'll get a scan and silence the doubts/fears," I thought. Managed to get a scan then and there.

Scan showed a perfect form but unfortunately no heartbeat. I broke. Had my two preschoolers with me in the room, but couldn't pretend everything was fine so I just allowed the tears to flow. I remember as I drove home how my heart screamed at God.

I thought He was so cruel – it seemed like He had played a practical joke on us by allowing us to see a strong heartbeat only two weeks before and now this! I told God He was truly mean. (At some point, probably after the D and C, I realized it was actually a blessing to have been given the opportunity to see baby's heartbeat and movement at the nuchal fold scan.)

This was my darkest moment. I was aware of how I needed to let myself experience all the emotions as deeply and as honestly as I knew how. It was a strange thing though, as all that time I knew deeply that God is good and was with me.

We prayed and fasted. As I was believing for a miracle, I needed food to nourish my baby, so I fasted from using the computer – no easy feat that's for sure.

Friday, April 4, 2008

Hoping the scan today would show a kicking baby. But it was not to be so.

While we don't understand the whys – we can truly say we sense the power of God as He carries us through this tragedy on almost the anniversary of our first miscarriage last year, with almost the same detail! So many people have been praying and believing with us, and I know it is also an answer to their prayers that Craig and I have a peace that passes all understanding.

Monday, April 7, 2008.

Had a D and C. I didn't want to go through the same experience as last year where I lost so much blood I almost needed a blood transfusion. After being discharged from the hospital in the late morning, I said to Craig we should go to the beach. I felt the fresh air would do me good and I wanted to spend some family time in the outdoors. I also thought it would be a good, reassuring time for our two boys.

Upon coming home, I decided to write a note to all our friends who had been praying for us:

Dear faithful friends and mighty prayer warriors!

Thank you everyone for your HUGE support of Craig and me in this past week as we went through a range of emotions – from peace and joy about our impending addition to the family, to shock and despair. We discovered that some time between twelve weeks when we had our first scan, and fifteen weeks, his/her heart had stopped beating.

We went from peace to anger and toddler tantrums at our Father, to a sense of belief for a miracle for life to be breathed back into what appeared to be a dead form. Though this belief was always there in the tiniest seed, it wavered to and fro but eventually, thanks to all of you believing with us and for us, it grew and grew. And so it was true, as a friend reminded me, that "our weakness makes room for God's strength." Your prayers and faith encouraged ours and God surely held on to us tightly when at times we felt too weak in despair and darkness. We have come to a sense of peace that indeed transcends all understanding even though the miracle we believed and hoped for was not to be, as we discovered last Friday.

We feel absolutely held in the loving arms of an all-knowing, all-good, all-powerful, all-merciful God.

The fact is that in the broken world in which we find ourselves, miscarriage and recurrent pregnancy loss is a reality. Medically, the cause of only 50% of recurrent loss is known and has a treatment plan – praise God for the human brain. Go medicine and technology! For the rest, "it's just one of those things that happens" is hardly a satisfactory or reassuring way to make sense of the situation. Our prayer is that for these couples, their despair would drive them towards life and relationship with God and trust in Him.

I want to affirm that God's strength is made perfect in our weakness. I keep believing for miracles. Faith is, after all, not to be based on experience, but on the Word of God. No doubt the accuser will remind us over and over again of our past experiences that did not demonstrate God's promise so I recognize that now. I am prepared and able to silence him and his accusations with God's Word.

Of course, Craig and I have a lot of WHYs for God. My prayer is that even as I seek Him for answers, I continue to be strengthened by, and to stand firm on His Word, not my experiences. And may he open our eyes to Jesus's promise in John 14:13-14 (NIV):"And I will do whatever you ask in my name, so that the Father may be glorified in the Son. You may ask me for anything in my name, and I will do it."

The question I have had to face on my faith journey is: "Can I trust God enough to place my life, my dreams, my everything in Him?" I choose to declare that: "Yes, I will! Yes, I do! With heart abandoned, in awe of the One who gives it all." (As the Hillsong song "I Stand" says).

We named this baby Jordan, as it has a spiritual connotation of 'Wise in Judgment" and the scriptural reference is Proverbs 21:30 (NCV), "There is no wisdom, understanding, or advice that can succeed against the Lord." Which is exactly how we feel. Also, Jordan is a gender-neutral name. While we believe that we lost another baby boy, we actually don't know for sure.

Nineteen months later…

September 24, 2009

Today as I sit here to write, I just want to shout hallelujah! My beautiful baby boy is almost three months old already. I haven't missed the poignancy of the fact that today would be Jordan's first birthday if he was birthed on his due date last year. And in three days time, when Joel will be three months old, it would be Zac's second birthday if he was born on his due date two years ago.

We never got to hold Zac and Jordan, we never got to see them grow and develop new skills like smiling, but we won't ever forget them. With each new skill Joel acquires, I will undoubtedly shed a tear or two at what we missed out on with Zac and Jordan. I will allow myself to feel the loss deeply, but knowing they are in the courts of heaven in the presence of Jesus, I will celebrate heartily for Joel as he reaches each milestone.

My pregnancy with Joel is a testimony to share another time; for now it is enough to say that God desires for us to walk in victory in Christ. There are lots of pearls to gain on our journey of trials. My prayer is that others will also grow in their relationship with Christ as they journey on, and know that His grace is indeed sufficient for them.

Dear Readers:

It is my heartfelt prayer that within these pages you have found comfort and hope and a part of your own journey. It is my desire that you will not feel alone as your travel this road; that you will know there are others out there who understand your pain, and weep with you.

And most importantly, it is my hope that you will know without a doubt that a loving Father in Heaven sees your pain and cares. He is not the creator of pain. He is the creator of life. By definition, He is love. He is able to penetrate even the deepest hurt and pour healing balm over your soul.

Jeremiah 31:13 (MSG) says that He will "convert their weeping into laughter, lavishing comfort, invading their grief with joy."

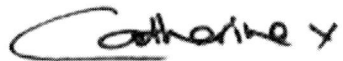

Glossary

Anemia - condition where patient has less than the normal amount of hemoglobin (red blood cells) in the blood therefore reducing the oxygen carrying capacity of the blood.

Blastocyst - a day 5 embryo.

D and C - gynecological procedure usually performed under general anesthesia, to open / dilate the cervix (entrance to the womb) and remove tissue eg. Miscarriage or to sample the lining tissue of the womb

Fragmented embryo - process where portions of the embryo cells have broken off and are separate from the nucleated portion of the cell; however fragmentation is quite common and successful pregnancies can occurr from these embryos.

GIFT - gamete intra fallopian tube transfer procedure performed before ovulation, egg removed from ovary via laparoscopy, mixed with washed sperm then sperm egg mixtures transferred by laparoscopy into the fallopian tubes where fertilization may then take place

ICSI - procedure in which sperm is injected directly into the egg to achieve fertilization

IUCD - intra uterine contraceptive device, a small T shaped plastic and metal device which sits inside the womb and provides a long lasting reversible method of contraception

IUI - the procedure in which prepared sperm is placed directly into the uterus for fertilization with the egg.

IVF - In Vitro Fertilization, procedure in which the ovaries are stimulated with hormone drugs, the eggs (oocytes) are collected, fertilization achieved either by allowing the sperm to penetrate the egg on its own or by using ICSI, the resulting embryo then returned to the uterus.

Laparoscopic surgery - surgical procedure involving the insertion of a telescopic surgical instrument through a small incision on the abdomen.

OHSS - ovarian hyper-stimulation syndrome, a complication of hormone stimulating drugs, most cases mild a small number are severe with abdominal pain and collection of fluid within body cavities.

PGD - pre implantation genetic diagnosis, procedure in which an embryo is tested to see if it is affected by the known genetic disorder carried by one of the parents.

The Bible - **(NIV)** The Bible New International Version
(MSG) The Message Bible
(NRSV) The Bible New Revised Standard Version
(NCV) The Bible New Century Version

Medical glossary provided by Dr Elizabeth Curr, Obstetrician & Gynecologist, Auckland City Hospital, New Zealand

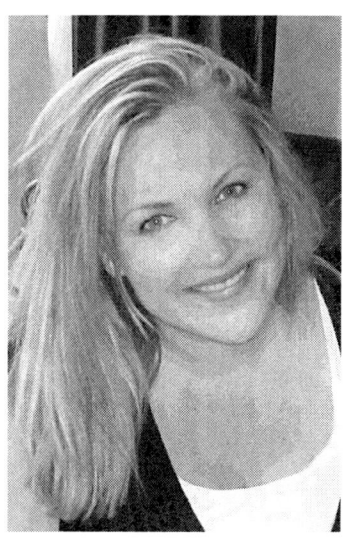

Catherine Sylvester was born in New Zealand and spent her first seventeen years there before living overseas in various countries and studying acting in Australia. Putting to use the skills she learned, she hosted various TV shows and a radio show.

Married to Julian since 2005, they absolutely love and delight in their girls, Estella and Skyler. As a family they are always keen for an adventure.

Since experiencing fertility issues and recurrent miscarriage, she has had the privilege of ministering to others who find themselves in a similar situation through Thursday's Babies which she founded in 2007. (www.thursdaysbabies.com)

It is Catherine's passion to share with others the restorative and redeeming love of a Father who forgives all, loves all and can do all things.

CPSIA information can be obtained at www.ICGtesting.com
Printed in the USA
LVOW091509290112

266072LV00022B/137/P